DEPRESSION IN CHILDHOOD:
DIAGNOSIS, TREATMENT, AND CONCEPTUAL MODELS

Depression in Childhood: Diagnosis, Treatment, and Conceptual Models

Edited by

Joy G. Schulterbrandt, M.S.

Chief, Center for Studies of Child and
Family Mental Health
National Institute of Mental Health
Rockville, Maryland

and

Allen Raskin, Ph.D.

Research Psychologist
Psychopharmacology Research Branch
National Institute of Mental Health
Rockville, Maryland

Raven Press ■ New York

Raven Press, 1140 Avenue of the Americas, New York, New York 10036

Raven Press, New York, 1977.

Made in the United States of America

International Standard Book Number 0-89004-147-4
Library of Congress Catalog Card Number 76-471-22

Foreword

Bertram S. Brown

Director, National Institute of Mental Health, Rockville, Maryland

These proceedings of the conference on Depression in Childhood represent the synthesis of many approaches to priority setting and program development taken over the years by the National Institute of Mental Health (NIMH).

The first, essential factor is, of course, the research capability of the Institute. More than 30 years ago, the National Mental Health Act authorized the establishment of an NIMH that would be triadic in structure, with major emphases in the areas of research, mental health services, and training and education of a mental health work force. While each of the programs has evolved to an extent separately and successfully—often in the face of challenging odds—research has been the keystone. The research endeavors of NIMH scientists and grantees have expanded the limits of our knowledge of human development as well as the more sharply defined areas of mental illness. This research yield has influenced dramatically the kinds of services, typified in the diverse programs of community mental health centers, that are available locally to more than 90 million Americans. It has had a marked effect on the design and content of training programs for professional and paraprofessional mental health workers. Perhaps the worth of the NIMH research effort is best measured by the extent of support it has claimed not only from the scientific community but from political bodies, citizen groups, and private individuals when its survival has been threatened by fiscal or other social pressures.

A second factor in the synthesis has been the priority set for child mental health by the Institute. Upon becoming Director of the Institute in 1970, I designated child mental health our foremost concern. The effect of this priority may be measured both quantitatively, in terms of numbers of grants and dollars expended with a primary focus on child mental health, and qualitatively, in terms of a gradual consciousness raising regarding the problems, needs, rights, and even the identities of children.

A third factor has been the strength and accomplishments of NIMH-supported projects in research on adult depression (without ignoring the invaluable contributions of scientists supported by other sources as well). The problem has elicited a tremendous response from the scientific community, making this life-crippling and sometimes fatal mental disorder among the most treatable and preventable of the severe mental illnesses.

An understanding of these factors is useful; it illustrates the timeliness of our current interest in depression in childhood. One immediate impetus to the conference on which this volume is based was a question posed to one of our scientists at a research briefing on depression sponsored by the NIMH for science newswriters. We realized the relative paucity of information in this area and agreed the time was ripe for the Institute, in its role as convener and catalyst, to attempt to coordinate the various facets of expertise necessary for designing research strategies.

Ms. Joy Schulterbrandt, Chief of the NIMH Center for Studies of Child and Family Mental Health, and Dr. Allen Raskin, NIMH Psychopharmacology Research Branch, were successful, as the listing of participants indicates, in identifying the needed expertise. The presentations speak for themselves. Collectively, the papers represent an early sortie into a field that has not been mapped out in a coordinated, multidisciplinary fashion.

The state-of-the-art of research on childhood depression is such that the first two sections of the volume might well be presented in reverse order. Innovative conceptual models will help resolve some of the discussions of symptom versus syndrome, of depression equivalencies and depressive behaviors among children. Conversely, refinement of the models cannot precede broader consensus on issues of definition and diagnosis.

We anticipate that the active involvement of the NIMH will enhance the vital and creative efforts of investigators now studying depression in children and also stimulate the interest of the scientific community and all child advocacy groups in this subject.

The more we contribute to and advance our culture socially and technologically, in areas ranging from evolving family lifestyles to increasingly sophisticated means of mass communication that bring the world—and its fantasies and foibles—into the home, the more we encroach on the once unquestioned phenomenon of a "happy childhood." Our responsibility is to protect and provide for the needs of the vulnerable children as we design the world they all will experience.

Preface

In contrast to the attention that has been focused on adult depression in the past 10 or 15 years, comparatively few investigators have been specifically identified with research in childhood depression. Difficulties in diagnosing depression in children or in operationally defining the symptoms of depression in children have been cited as major obstacles to clinical investigations in this field. However, some recent developments in this area attracted our attention and led to the decision to convene a conference on childhood depression in Washington, D.C., on September 19–20, 1975. The chapters in this volume are based on the papers and discussions of these papers presented at the conference. The conference itself was sponsored by the Center for Studies of Child and Family Mental Health of the National Institute, of Mental Health (NIMH).

Utilizing different techniques and approaches a number of investigators, including Drs. Malmquist, Cytryn, and Kovacs and Beck, have attempted to elucidate the major symptoms of depression in children. Some of these individuals are also in the process of developing inventories for rating depression in children. One aim of the conference was to bring participants up to date on these developments, to review critically existing approaches for assessing depression in children, and to suggest modifications and new approaches for establishing the presence and severity of depression in children. A related aim was to obtain from participants some estimates on the magnitude of the problem, i.e., how prevalent is depression in children?

We had several additional goals. One was to examine the treatment of depression in children, and in particular the use of antidepressant drugs in this age group. How frequently are these drugs prescribed and do they work? It was also deemed desirable to include some of the more recent and provocative results with animals and children that provide a conceptual or theoretical basis for the onset of depression in children and adults. Included in this category are Dr. McKinney's studies on the effects of maternal separation in monkeys and Dr. Watson's studies on perception of control in young infants. Yet a further aim was to provide guidelines for the NIMH on future research and development needs in this area, and recommendations of the subcommittees formed for this purpose are included as appendix in this volume.

When the conference was first conceived it was structured principally as a working and planning meeting for selected investigators with similar interests in three broad areas: the definition and diagnosis of depression in children, the treatment of depression in children, and models for conceptualizing depression in children. However, it soon became apparent that the formal papers and the discussions of these papers deserved wider distribution and would interest all professionals who work with emotionally disturbed children, including the practicing clinician and the researcher. We hope you share this view.

Joy G. Schulterbrandt
Allen Raskin
Editors

Acknowledgments

We are grateful to the conference participants whose special knowledge about children is reflected in the quality of the articles in this book. Their expert knowledge of the state-of-the-art has been extremely valuable to us in planning future directions and emphases in our exploration of depression in young children.

In planning the conference on which this volume is based, a number of persons from within the National Institute of Mental Health gave generously of their professional expertise, experience, and time. Special mention, however, must go to Drs. Louis A. Wienckowski, David Pearl, and Martin Katz of the Division of Extramural Research Programs, National Institute of Mental Health, and Dr. Stephen P. Hersh, Office of the Director, National Institute of Mental Health, for their consultation in selecting the highly qualified participants.

Finally, thanks are also in order to Mrs. Mary Povich, Mrs. Diane Cheslosky, Mrs. Selma Greenhouse, and Mrs. El-Marie Hamilton, all of the National Institute of Mental Health, for their excellent secretarial assistance and for smoothly coordinating services for the conference.

Joy G. Schulterbrandt
Allen Raskin
Editors

Contents

Participants and Contributors

E. James Anthony, M.D.
*Director, Eliot Division of Child
Psychiatry
Washington University School of
Medicine
St. Louis, Missouri 63130*

G. LaVonne Brown, M.D.
*Medical Officer
Division of Clinical and Behavioral
Research
Adult Psychiatry Branch
National Institutes of Health
Bethesda, Maryland 20014*

William E. Bunney, M.D.
*Chief, Adult Psychiatry Branch
National Institutes of Health
Bethesda, Maryland 20014*

C. Keith Conners, Ph.D.
*Associate Professor of Psychiatry
Western Psychiatric Institute and
Clinics
University of Pittsburgh School of
Medicine
Pittsburgh, Pennsylvania 15261*

Leon Cytryn, Ph.D.
*Medical Officer
Unit on Childhood Mental Illness
Adult Psychiatry Branch
National Institutes of Health
Bethesda, Maryland 20014*

Carol S. Dweck, Ph.D.
*Department of Psychology
University of Illinois
Urbana, Illinois 61820*

Rachel Gittelman-Klein, Ph.D.
*Director, Child Development Clinic
Department of Psychiatry
Long Island Jewish-Hillside Medical
Center
Glen Oaks, New York 11004*

Stephen P. Hersh, M.D.
*Assistant Director for Children and
Youth
National Institute of Mental Health
Rockville, Maryland 20014*

Martin M. Katz, Ph.D.
*Chief, Clinical Research Branch
Division of Extramural Research
Programs
National Institute of Mental Health
Rockville, Maryland 20014*

Maria Kovacs, Ph.D.
*University of Pennsylvania Medical
School
Philadelphia General Hospital
Philadelphia, Pennsylvania 19104*

Monroe Lefkowitz, Ph.D.
*New York State Department of Mental
Hygiene
Albany, New York 12208*

Ben Z. Locke, M.S.P.H.
*Acting Chief, Center for Epidemiologic
Studies
Division of Biometry and Epidemiology
National Institute of Mental Health
Rockville, Maryland 20014*

Carl P. Malmquist, M.D.
*Professor, Law School and Department
of Criminal Justice
University of Minnesota
Minneapolis, Minnesota 55455*

William T. McKinney, M.D.
*Chairman, Department of Psychiatry
University Hospital
Madison, Wisconsin 53706*

Anthony Nowels, M.D.
*Acting Director, Department of Child
Psychiatry
Department of Psychiatry
University of Miami School of Medicine
Miami, Florida 33124*

Judith L. Rapoport, M.D.
Department of Pediatrics
Georgetown University Hospital
Washington, D.C. 20007

Allen Raskin, Ph.D.
Research Psychologist
Psychopharmacology Research Branch
National Institute of Mental Health
Rockville, Maryland 20857

Natalie Reatig, B.A.
Social Science Analyst
Clinical Studies Section
National Institute of Mental Health
Rockville, Maryland 20014

Joy G. Schulterbrandt, M.S.
Chief, Center for Studies of Child and
    Family Mental Health
National Institute of Mental Health
Rockville, Maryland 20014

John S. Watson, Ph.D.
Associate Professor of Psychology
Department of Psychology
University of California
Berkeley, California 94720

Definition, Diagnosis, and Treatment

Depression in Childhood: Diagnosis, Treatment, and Conceptual Models, edited by J. G. Schulter-brandt and A. Raskin. Raven Press, New York, 1977.

An Empirical-Clinical Approach Toward a Definition of Childhood Depression

Maria Kovacs and Aaron T. Beck

Department of Psychiatry, University of Pennsylvania, Philadelphia, Pennsylvania 19104

INTRODUCTION

In our extensive work with depressed adults, we have pursued a number of objectives over the past 20 years. We have described and delineated crucial symptoms of the adult depressive syndromes. We have contributed to the understanding, classification, and treatment of depressive states. We have consistently stressed the need for description, measurement, and empirical investigations as steps necessary for ultimate theoretical conceptualization. Over the years, one of us (A.T.B.) has extensively contributed to a more systematic understanding of the symptom cluster that makes up the adult depressive syndrome, has constructed and validated a screening and diagnostic instrument that also became an efficient research tool, and has contributed toward understanding the psychology of depressive syndromes.

In light of our extensive findings on adult depressives, we became interested in examining the phenomena of depression in children. One of our first steps was to examine the current clinical and empirical literature in this area for guidelines about symptom clusters considered characteristic of childhood depression.

The distinction must be made firmly between depression as a sad, despondent mood, and depression as a clinical syndrome (a collection of symptoms). Our past experience with adult depressives consistently indicated that depression as psychopathology is definitely a syndrome, and not just a dysphoric mood state. The concept of a depressive syndrome in adults is debated by few who work in clinical settings. It is further supported by various empirical scales and inventories that quantify the severity of adult depression (e.g., Zung Depression Inventory, Hamilton Rating Scale for Depression, Raskin Depression Scale).

In going into a relatively novel area, we have always started with what is "known." We essentially looked for syndrome descriptions, since it is known that adult depression, as psychopathology, exists as a syndrome, and since we could think of no *a priori* evidence that a syndrome should not be evident in childhood depression.

Our initial perusal of the literature disclosed a prevalent opinion that among children under 5 or 6 years of age, depressive disorders either do not exist or are exceedingly difficult to recognize. Thus, we decided to concentrate on clinical and empirical publications focused on children from the ages of 6 to 7 years up to early adolescence. Our decision was reinforced by the findings of Piaget and his co-workers (Ginsburg and Opper, 1969) that language, as a vehicle for communicating information, becomes apparent only around the age of 7. We felt it important to look at studies dealing with children who can use language to communicate, since among adults the verbal communication of self-assessment is a decisive factor in assessing presence or absence of depression.

A SELECTED REVIEW OF RELEVANT LITERATURE

Descriptions of childhood depressive disorders seem to represent two general, somewhat overlapping viewpoints: (1) that childhood depressive disorders and adult syndromes have a number of similarities, but also have some additional unique, *overt* features, and (2) that childhood depressive disorders are different from adult syndromes and are *not* manifest in *overt* depressive symptoms.

The first viewpoint is exemplified by Ling, Oftedal, and Weinberg (1970) in a study designed to identify and define depressive illness in youngsters. These investigators employed some of the well-established clinical characteristics of adult depression in combination with factors more readily observable in children (Table 1). A child was considered depressed if he fulfilled any four of the criteria listed in Table 1 and apparently had no other clear-cut psychiatric illness. In a sample of 25 children, aged 4 to 16, who presented to neurology services with severe headaches, 10 had a depressive disorder that could be recognized by the criteria specified. The authors noted that mood change, social withdrawal, and self-depreciation were the most common symptoms. Sleep disturbance, decreased school performance, and various somatic complaints were also evident in 7 of the 10 depressed children.

Weinberg, Rutman, Sullivan, Penick, and Dietz (1973) examined a sample of 72 children, aged 6 years 6 months to 12 years 8 months (50 boys and 22 girls) who were referred to an educational diagnostic center. Among other things, they sought to determine what portion of the children suffered from depression "possibly as a primary entity." They essentially used the symptom list of Ling et al. (1970). In order to be diagnosed as depressed, a child had to have *both* dysphoric mood and self-deprecatory ideation, and two or more of the additional eight symptoms (Table 1). Moreover, the symptoms had to have been present for more than 1 month.

Weinberg et al. (1973) reported that 42 of the 72 children met these criteria (12 girls and 30 boys). All the depressed children presented with school and/or behavior problems, and the parents were generally unable to relate the behavioral change to specific environmental events. The most common manifestations of depression were agitated behavior, crying, moodiness, often with sleep disturbance and/or somatic complaints; activity level varied from decreased activity to hyperactivity. Fifteen children reported death wishes, and three had attempted suicide. Compared to a group of nondepressed children, none of whom had more than 4 symptoms, 57% of the depressed children had 7 or more of the 10 symptoms listed in Table 1. No differences were found in sex, age, grade, and tested IQ.

A recent paper by McConville, Boag, and Purohit (1973) describes three types of childhood depression in a group of 6- to 13-year-old inpatients. Based on the daily entries of trained child care workers and other staff, the authors identified 75 children for whom the therapeutic group described depression as a "prime target symptom." The records of these children were then examined for reference to "depressive items."

Fifteen depressive items were selected on the grounds of clinical frequency (Table 1). Apparently based on some clustering of items, the authors described three types of childhood depression: (1) The *affectual depression* group was characterized by phenomena such as expressions of sadness and helplessness as well as occasional hopelessness, (2) The *negative self-esteem depression* group included children in whom "thoughts-feelings" about depression predominated, seemingly based on fixed ideas of negative self-esteem including worthlessness, being unloved, and being used by other people, (3) The *guilt depression* group included a rather small number of children who felt that they were "wicked" and that they should be dead or killed, either because of essential badness or so that they might be reunited with a dead person.

Affectual depression was most common among 6- to 8-year-olds; negative self-esteem depression was more frequent after the age of 8 and remained at a relatively high level even after age 11; guilt depression became more frequent after age 11 even though it was still relatively uncommon.

Eva Frommer has been one of the most fervent advocates of the existence of overt depression in childhood. However, like a number of other authors, she also points out that *presenting complaints* are most commonly of a nonspecific, somatic nature. In order to bring out the distinguishing features of juvenile depressive illness, she compared 74 children who were suffering from a neurotic disorder (including some depressive features) to a group of 190 depressed youngsters (Frommer, 1968).

According to Frommer (1968), five symptoms *significantly* differentiate the

TABLE 1. *Characteristics of childhood depressive disorders*

Publication	Characteristic depressive features, symptoms	
Ling, Oftedal, and Weinberg, 1970	1. Significant mood change 2. Social withdrawal 3. Increasingly poor performance in school 4. Sleep disturbances 5. Aggressive behavior not previously present 6. Self-depreciation and beliefs of persecution 7. Lack of energy 8. Somatic complaints other than headaches 9. School phobia 10. Weight loss and anorexia Note: emphasis was placed on recent changes in behavior.	
Weinberg, Rutman, Sullivan, Penick, and Dietz, 1973	1. Dysphoric mood 2. Self-deprecatory ideation 3. Aggressive behavior 4. Sleep disturbance 5. Change in school performance 6. Diminished socialization 7. Change in attitude toward school 8. Somatic complaints 9. Loss of usual energy 10. Unusual change in appetite and/or weight Note: emphasis was placed on recent changes in behavior.	
McConville, Boag, and Purohit, 1973	1. Sadness 2. Helplessness 3. Loneliness 4. Feelings of loss 5. Unspecified feelings of being bad 6. Negative self-esteem 7. Feelings of being unable to help 8. Unable to do things for others 9. Inability to be liked 10. Expectations of being used 11. Feelings that the situation will not change 12. Feelings of being wicked 13. Feelings of being hated because of actions 14. Feelings of being justly punished 15. Suicidal ideation	
Frommer, 1968	1. Irritability 2. Weepiness 3. Complaint of depression 4. Tension and explosiveness	5. Moodiness 6. Enuresis 7. Encopresis
Arajärvi and Huttunen, 1972	1. Inhibition 2. Poor self-confidence 3. Passivity 4. Lack of spontaneous activity	5. Encopresis 6. Enuresis
Poznanski and Zrull, 1970 ("affective depression")	1. Sad, unhappy, and/or depressed 2. Excessive self-criticism 3. Feelings of inadequacy 4. Difficulty sleeping 5. Excessive concerns about death	

TABLE 1. *Characteristics of childhood depressive disorders (continued)*

Publication	Characteristic depressive features, symptoms
Vranješević Radojičić, Bumbaširević, and Todorović, 1972	1. Is sad, unhappy, apt to cry 2. Is rejected and unloved 3. Retreats, loses interest in objects and situations previously interested in 4. May be preoccupied with death or suicidal thoughts 5. Has neurovegetative symptoms
Kuhn and Kuhn, 1972	1. Morning tiredness 2. Poor school performance 3. Sleep problems 4. Inhibition 5. Disturbance in mental activity (concentration) 6. Dissatisfaction 7. Weepiness 8. Sensitivity
Connell, 1972	1. Negative self-concept 2. Irritability 3. Weeps frequently 4. Behavioral change (anergic-restless) 5. Feels rejected 6. Social withdrawal 7. Morbid ideas 8. Suicide 9. Headache 10. Nausea 11. Appetite loss 12. Abdominal pain 13. Enuresis/encopresis 14. Sleep disturbance 15. Compensatory symptoms (bulimia, stealing) 16. Antisocial behavior (negativism, destructive acts, fire setting) 17. Anxiety, hypochrondriasis

depressed from the neurotic children (Table 1). Based on two additional symptoms (enuresis and encopresis), Frommer then grouped 264 depressed youngsters, ages 3 to 16, into three types who allegedly show differing "clinical patterns" and "treatment needs." (1) The *enuretic and/or encopretic depressives:* these childrens' most common symptoms were moodiness, weepiness, immaturity, as well as hostile and antisocial behavior. Moreover, children in this group had a depressive disorder that was often of long standing. (2) Children with *uncomplicated depression:* among these children, irritability, weepiness, a tendency to recurrent explosions of temper and misery, often with no adequate explanation, were characteristic features. In addition, these youngsters more frequently had difficulty in going to sleep than the other groups and often reported sleep disturbances such as nightmares, sleepwalking, and talking in sleep. (3) Children with a *depressive phobic anxiety state:* although these children also had "typical depressive symptoms, such as weepiness, tension, and irritability" they are described as "considerably less moody and more apathetic" than the other groups. Increasing abdominal pain was most characteristically present in this group. In addition to the above, Frommer also lists various other characteristics that highlight the differential "clinical patterns," namely premorbid personality traits and family factors.

Arajärvi and Huttunen (1972) also described encopresis and enuresis as symptoms of depression in a series of 44 children, aged 5 to 12. In addition to encopresis and enuresis, inhibition, poor self-confidence, passivity, submissiveness, and lack of spontaneous activity were listed as symptoms of childhood depression.

In a clinically oriented study, Poznanski and Zrull (1970) set out to describe "affective depression" in children. The charts of 1,788 children, up to age 12, were examined for the following elements: description of the child as sad, unhappy, and showing excessive self-criticism, feelings of inadequacy, difficulty in sleeping, and excessive concerns about death. For each chart, the examiners also "rated" the severity or predominance of depression. Out of 66 children, aged 7 to 12, rated "severe" or "predominant," only 10 had the necessary description of "affective depression."

Based on the records selected, Poznanski and Zrull (1970) claimed that "the most frequent disturbance seen within the depressive symptomatology was a negative self image." The children often described themselves as "mean," "stupid," and "punk kid." In line with other papers cited above, Poznanski and Zrull also noted that difficulty in handling aggression was the most frequent symptomatic behavior which initiated *referral.*

Vranješević, Radojičić, Bumbaširević, and Todorović (1972) described depressed children in terms that come close to those describing the adult syndrome (Table 1): negative affect, rejection, withdrawal and diminished interest, preoccupation with death or suicidal thoughts, and neurovegetative symptoms. They add, however, that in the older child it may not be uncommon "to run away" from such unpleasant feelings and show delinquent or antisocial behavior.

A study by Kuhn and Kuhn (1972) on the imipramine treatment of 100 depressed children found "morning tiredness" to be the "cardinal symptom." Their list of additional symptoms also parallels elements of the adult depressive syndrome (Table 1).

Numerous other writers have described childhood depression in ways that closely resemble the adult syndrome. For instance, Krakowski (1970) focuses on lowered self-esteem as a consequence of loss. He notes that almost all the symptoms of the adult syndrome described by Beck (1967) are seen in children "but their character is somewhat different."

Connell's (1972) pilot study on the nature of childhood depression notes that psychosomatic or behavioral *complaints* among children often mask the underlying affective disturbance. Connell used eight standard pediatric psychiatric texts as well as a paper by Frommer to extract three patterns of symptoms that indicate depression in childhood (Table 1): (1) symptoms associated with change in affect (symptoms 1 through 8); (2) pathophysiological symptoms (symptoms 9 through 14); and (3) other compensatory symptoms (symptoms 15 through 17).

In the Connell study, there were 20 children who had been referred because of mood disturbance. Only those children whose parents described them as persistently unhappy or depressed were selected. Notably, 6 of the 20 index children presented with physical symptoms and another 6 with school or behavioral difficulties. A control group of 12 children was drawn from the general hospital population. Based on the syndromes extracted from the texts, a symptom score of 18 was derived. The average symptom score for the depressed children was 10.6 compared to the controls whose score was 2.6. The author concludes that although the index children suffered from a mood disturbance, a chief characteristic was "the prominence of somatic symptoms and antisocial behavior." She then concludes that in many cases "the depression could be regarded as masked, or virtually ignored."

Glaser has been one of the strongest proponents of the viewpoint that childhood depressive disorders differ from adult syndromes. Glaser (1968) has taken the position that depression in youngsters is generally "masked" by symptoms not readily identifiable with this condition. His concept of masked depression consists of two contentions: (1) the child should present with symptoms not usually associated with depression, and (2) "there should be sufficient evidence that the patient's psychopathology features depressive elements." He defines depressive elements in terms of negative self-evaluation (Table 2) as well as rejection by others (either self-expressed or assessed by the clinician in the interview situation). He adds that these elements should be somewhat unwarranted and not correspond to the child's actual life situation.

According to Glaser, in older children and adolescents the following symptom pictures may indicate or mask an "underlying depression": (1) behavioral problems and delinquent behavior; (2) psychoneurotic reactions; and (3) psychophysiologic reactions (Table 2). Moreover, the concealed depressive elements are *not* identical to the "classic" entity of depression nor to the self-limited depressive episodes known in adult psychiatry. However, Glaser does not delineate clearly what he really means by this statement.

In his 1962 paper, Toolan takes the position that although "overt manifestations of depression are rare in children and adolescents, depressive feelings and depressive equivalents are commonly encountered." He states that the adult clinical picture of depression—namely, retardation in mental and physical activity, insomnia, feelings of depression, apathy, worthlessness, and nihilism as well as suicidal preoccupations—is rarely encountered in children and adolescents. According to Toolan, depressive feelings in the growing child

TABLE 2. *Characteristics of masked depressive disorders in childhood*

Publication	Masking symptoms depressive equivalents	Depressive symptoms
Glaser, 1968	1. Temper tantrums, disobedience, truancy, running away, delinquent behavior 2. School phobia, failure to achieve in school, other psychoneurotic reactions 3. Psychophysiologic reactions	1. Feelings of inadequacy 2. Worthlessness 3. Low self-esteem 4. Helplessness and hopelessness 5. Rejection by others 6. Isolation
Toolan, 1962	1. Temper tantrums 2. Disobedience 3. Truancy 4. Running away from home 5. Accident proneness 6. Masochism 7. Self-destructive behavior 8. Boredom 9. Restlessness 10. Sexual acting out	1. Withdrawal 2. Apathy 3. "Depressive feelings" 4. Feeling unloved, unwanted 5. Preoccupation with death and injury (in dreams), emptiness
Cytryn and McKnew, 1974	1. Hyperactivity 2. Aggressiveness 3. School failure 4. Delinquency	1. Negative fantasy and dream content: themes of mistreatment, thwarting, blame, criticism, loss, injury, death,

	5. Psychosomatic symptoms	suicide 2. Hopelessness, helplessness, guilt, worthlessness, being unloved (verbally expressed) 3. Motor retardation, sad faces and posture, appetite and sleep disturbance
Bakwin, 1972	1. Acting out 2. Poor school performance 3. Aggressive behavior 4. Irritability	1. Sadness and unhappiness 2. Loss of self-esteem 3. Dissatisfaction with the world 4. Decreased ability to get fun out of things 5. Moping 6. Listlessness, apathy, 7. Spiritlessness, dejection 8. Reduced interest in school work
Renshaw, 1974	1. Angry outbursts 2. School avoidance 3. Physical complaints (abdominal pains, headaches, recurrent vomiting) 4. Whining and whimpering 5. Phobias 6. Fire setting 7. Running away	1. Feelings of sorrow, tearfulness 2. Suicide attempts 3. Brooding 4. Apathy 5. Preoccupations with morbidity 6. Inactivity 7. Sleep and appetite disturbance 8. Supersensitivity 9. Withdrawal

are displaced by behavioral problems (Table 2). The youngster is convinced that he is "bad, evil, and unacceptable," and such feelings lead him into antisocial behavior. Thus, Toolan feels that all of the behavioral symptoms he describes "should be considered as evidence of depression." He notes that the overt depressive themes may be uncovered in fantasies and dreams and through responses to projective tests.

Cytryn and McKnew (1974) are of the opinion that "masked depressive reaction" is the most common form of depression in children, and that depressive mood and behavior are rare. They claim that depression in children is manifested in three ways: (1) fantasy or dream content, (2) verbal expression, and (3) mood and behavior (Table 2). Signs of masked depression include hyperactivity, aggressiveness, school failure, delinquency, and psychosomatic symptoms. Cytryn and McKnew also state that the underlying depression is inferred mostly from "periodic displays of a purely depressive picture and depressive themes on projective tests." Moreover, in most serious cases, the child's thinking is also affected by feelings of despair and hopelessness and, in the severe form, by suicidal thoughts. However, these authors also note that among latency-age children there is a group that does tend to present a more clearly identifiable depressive syndrome (which includes sad affect, social withdrawal, hopelessness, helplessness, psychomotor retardation, anxiety, as well as school and social failure, sleep and feeding disturbances, and suicidal ideas).

Bakwin (1972) also takes the position that depression in children is often masked by other behavioral manifestations such as acting out, poor school performance, aggressive behavior, and irritability. However, he also notes that "loss of self-esteem" is a prominent symptom of depressed children: the "child regards himself as a failure—a jerk, a flop." In addition to the other core symptoms of depression (i.e., the appearance of sadness and unhappiness), there are frequent somatic and other complaints (Table 2). Headaches and poor appetite may be presenting symptoms.

Numerous other authors essentially subscribe to the view that at various phases of development, depression is masked or becomes manifest in depressive equivalents. Examples are Renshaw (1974) who claims, in addition to the symptoms noted by others, that fire setting is a means of acting out childhood depression (Table 2) and Malmquist (1972) who lists depressive equivalents (including anorexia nervosa and obesity syndromes) in his tentative classification of childhood depressive phenomena.

COMMENTS ON THE LITERATURE

The literature reviewed above has some remarkable components. First, despite the insistence that childhood depressive disorders and the adult syndromes are dissimilar, we are struck by the similarities.

Beck (1967) has grouped symptoms of the adult depressive syndrome into

Item # 3471100101018847   routed to LISTX.

four categories: (1) affective changes, (2) cognitive changes, (3) motivational changes, and (4) vegetative and psychomotor disturbances. A perusal of Tables 1 and 2 shows *all* the symptoms listed under Beck's four categories, although perhaps phrased in different ways. As Table 1 indicates, all the studies reviewed agree that childhood depression involves some type of cognitive change in the negative direction, and most studies list attitudinal-motivational changes and disturbances in vegetative and psychomotor functions. However, the studies do not all put a uniform emphasis on dysphoric mood, *per se,* as a primary symptom of childhood depression.

An essentially similar picture is obtained by examining Table 2. As a matter of fact, both the data in Table 2 and the corresponding publications described suggest that the term "masked" depression may be misleading and unnecessary. Proponents of the concept of masked depression make it clear that masked depression cannot be diagnosed without proof of depression. Moreover, many of the symptoms specified as masking depression are essentially nothing more than presenting complaints.

We know from adult clinical practice that patients often present with either nonspecific somatic complaints or general malaise. Yet we do not refer to such adult presenting complaints as "masking" depression. We view them either as "somatizations" or as culturally accepted ways of construing or manifesting psychological discomfort. Consequently, concepts such as masked depression in childhood are unnecessary. The concept seems to have no clinical or heuristic significance and essentially signifies: (1) events that initiate referral, or (2) manifestations of a psychological disturbance acceptable or appropriate to that age category.

DESCRIPTION AND ASSESSMENT OF CHILDHOOD DEPRESSION

Introduction

As noted above, the literature generally indicates that in children some phenomena exist that are akin to the depressive syndrome in adults. Moreover, the various papers suggest that *description* of these phenomena is feasible. However, there is a considerable need to standardize the description and to delineate its domain.

A relatively standardized, agreed-on description of the characteristics of childhood depression is a necessary first step in bringing clarity to the field. Description and measurement of phenomena then lend themselves to classification schemas. Subsequent to that, efforts may be addressed to the investigation of etiology and the unique characteristics of the classified phenomena, variables that may eventually contribute to some theoretical schema— namely, onset and course and psychological, interpersonal, and biochemical characteristics.

A Preliminary Survey

Our extensive work with depressed adults led to the development of the Beck Depression Inventory (BDI), which taps and quantifies the varied aspects of the adult depressive syndrome. The BDI consists of 21 items (Beck, 1967, 1972; Beck and Beamesderfer, 1974) that assess the presence and severity of affective, cognitive, motivational, vegetative, and psychomotor components of depression. It has been employed with diverse groups of patients as well as with normal populations. Its reliability and validity on adult samples have been repeatedly confirmed (Beck and Beamesderfer, 1974).

Each BDI item consists of four choices, rated in severity from 0 to 3. Thus, the possible range of BDI scores is from 0 to 63. The following cutoff scores have been reported for psychiatric samples:

0–9——no depression   16–23   ——moderate depression
10–15——mild depression   24–above——severe depression

A short version of the BDI has also been developed (Beck and Beck, 1972; Beck, Rial, and Rickels, 1974). The short version consists of the 13 items that correlated highest with total long BDI scores. The possible score range for the short BDI is 0 to 26. Cutoff scores for psychiatric populations are as follows:

0–4——no depression   8–15   ——moderate depression
5–7——mild depression   16–above——severe depression

Because of the reported validity and reliability of the BDI to assess depressive phenomena among adults, we were interested in its possible applicability to children. Thus, our first question was: *Is there any evidence that children will endorse BDI items similar to those endorsed by adults or will endorse them in a similar way?*

Method

One of our collaborators administered the short BDI to a sample of 63 children in the 7th and 8th grades of a parochial school in suburban Philadelphia (Albert, 1973; Albert and Beck, 1975). The sample consisted of 36 boys and 27 girls, whose ages ranged from 11 years 2 months to 15 years 1 month. The BDI was administered in a group (classroom) setting. In addition to administering the BDI, Albert constructed six "adjustment items" that related to school, social, and family adjustment, as well as satisfaction with school performance. Teacher evaluations of the students' classroom performance were also obtained.

Results

For the total sample, Albert obtained an $\bar{X}$ BDI score of 7.06, with a range of 0 to 24. The mean BDI score was 6.23 for the 7th grade and 7.95 for the 8th grade. Girls tended to score higher than the boys, especially in the 8th grade. Among adult samples, a score of 7 is the upper limit of the "mildly depressed" category. If we tentatively compare the score distribution with the cutoff ranges established for adults, we find that approximately 33% of the sample falls into the "moderate" to "severe depression" category (scores 8 to 16+; $N=23$). Two of the 23 subjects (3%) had scores of 16 or above.

One of the interesting and promising aspects of this survey was the item choices endorsed that indicate degrees of mild to serious concerns in the area tapped, in other words, item choices greater than 0 (Table 3). In Table 3, the data for the items are presented as $\overline{X}$ scores, as well as the percentage of subjects who endorsed item choices of 1 or above. Since score distributions per item were rather skewed, the last column in Table 3 is worthy of note. For example, a surprising 33% of the subjects endorsed choices on the self-harm item, which indicates degrees of suicidal ideation.

Over 50% of the sample apparently had concerns about self-dislike, work difficulty, dissatisfaction, and indecisiveness. Between 29% and 49% of the sample had thoughts concerning sense of failure, fatigability, self-image change, guilt, anorexia, social withdrawal, self-harm, pessimism, and sadness.

Moreover, Albert reported that all the students whose classroom performance was rated by the teachers as "excellent" had "low" BDI scores, whereas all the students rated as "poor" had "high" BDI scores. The correlation between BDI scores and sum of the six adjustment items was 0.62 in the 7th grade and 0.60 in the 8th grade. Thus, it appears that self-reported problems in adjustment (namely, loneliness, dislike of school and poor school performance, not having friends, and not getting along with others as well as with family) correlate with BDI scores.

TABLE 3. *Percentage of subjects who endorsed BDI item choices greater than "0" (N = 63)*

BDI item	$\overline{X}$ item score	Endorsed choices 1, 2, or 3 (%)
Sadness	0.37	29
Pessimism	0.41	32
Sense of failure	0.64	48
Dissatisfaction	0.70	56
Guilt	0.44	38
Self-dislike	0.71	60
Self-harm	0.38	33
Social withdrawal	0.38	35
Indecisiveness	0.75	51
Self-image change	0.62	41
Work difficulty	0.66	57
Fatigability	0.48	44
Anorexia	0.43	37

From Albert, 1973.

The self-reported phenomenology of some of these youngsters seemed to resemble the picture obtained from clinically depressed adults. Naturally, we wondered if the pictures actually represented the same thing. It seemed unlikely that items endorsed in some degree by a large proportion of the students would reflect "genuine" depression. A more parsimonious explanation would be that those items by themselves might tap developmental issues in this age group.

To get a clearer idea of whether the items actually cluster the way they do in adult depressive samples, we did a separate tabulation for children whose total BDI score fell into "moderate-severe" adult depression range. Table 4 presents the percentage of these subjects who endorsed item choices that indicate discomfort in the symptom area tapped. As the data in Table 4 indicate, among these ostensibly depressed youngsters we are dealing with a syndrome not unlike that found in adult depressions.

The above-reviewed literature suggests that the presence of dysphoric mood may characterize a subcategory of childhood depressives. Thus, we attempted an item breakdown for children who denied any sadness versus those who admitted to some degree of dysphoric mood. Unfortunately, the uneven numbers (9 versus 14) made any comparisons unfeasible and misleading.

In spite of the promising results, we were still concerned whether the picture we obtained represented the same syndrome as in adults. Consequently, we embarked on a pilot study to establish the validity of the BDI as a measure of depression among children. As of now, we have no conclusive data, but the steps taken so far will be described.

TABLE 4. *Percentage of moderately to severely depressed subjects who endorsed BDI item choices greater than "0" (N = 23)*

BDI item	Endorsed choices 1, 2, or 3 (%)
Sadness	60
Pessimism	42
Sense of failure	81
Dissatisfaction	69
Guilt	56
Self-dislike	90
Self-harm	52
Social withdrawal	42
Indecisiveness	72
Self-image change	64
Work difficulty	64
Fatigability	55
Anorexia	68

Pilot Study on a Psychiatric Sample

The Philadelphia Child Guidance Clinic, which is affiliated with the Department of Psychiatry at the University of Pennsylvania School of Medicine, agreed to cooperate with us in this pilot investigation. Our initial aims were: (1) to modify the format of the BDI for use with children, (2) to validate this instrument for use with children, and (3) to assess, eventually, the prevalence of depressive symptomatology among youngsters. We decided to work with children between the ages of 10 and 15, who were inpatients or day care patients.

Step 1. Four children, between the ages of 11 and 15, who were about to be discharged from the Center, assisted in modifying the format of the BDI. Each child was individually asked for feedback as to how to put the item choices in a format that would be "clear to kids." This revision of the 21-item BDI was then further tested.

The final childhood version of the BDI retains the original item content and topic; only some of the words or phraseology were changed into the language of 10- to 15-year-olds. It should be noted that we originally deleted the item on sexual interest and substituted an item on loneliness. The tentative Childhood Depression Inventory (CDI) was then administered individually to seven additional children, aged 9 to 15. The total scores obtained were as follows: 0, 6, 10, 12, 18, 20, and 46. An examination of the individual protocols indicated that the children did not have a response bias. Of the five children with scores of 10 or above, two endorsed the item on sadness and showed some degree of pessimism and self-blame.

Step 2. In order to validate the CDI, we first needed to obtain clinical agreement in diagnosing depression. We invited a number of clinicians to discuss our diagnostic criteria. In this phase of the pilot study, Dr. Eliot Gursky and Mrs. Nila Betof of the Child Guidance Clinic were helpful.

We decided not to use the concept of depressive equivalents, since we had difficulty agreeing on symptoms. We then interviewed a number of children. After the interview we used a scale of 0 (none) to 8 (severe) to give our individual ratings of the overall severity of depression:

0 ——no depression	5–6——moderate depression
1–2——minimal depression	7–8——severe depression
3–4——mild depression	

We finally established that we were all following the same criteria in rating depression, and we tended to agree within two points on the ratings on overall severity. The next phase of the study will be undertaken shortly, namely: determination of inter-rater agreement and validation of CDI against clinical ratings. We have developed a Diagnostic Statement on which the clinicians rate the following items:

1. *Depression*—Overall.
2. *Emotional indices of depression*—Low mood, crying, loneliness, apathy, loss of attachment.
3. *Cognitive indices of depression*—Negative self-view, guilt, self-blame, self-criticism, indecisiveness, hopelessness, negative expectations (pessimism), and inability to fulfill parents' expectations.
4. *Motivational indices of depression*—Avoidance, escapism, withdrawal wishes, suicidal ideation, decreased motivation, increased dependency.
5. *Vegetative–physical indices of depression*—Appetite disturbance, sleep disturbance, increased tiredness.
6. *Objective observable behavior at interview*—Sad face and looks, dejected actions, crying, tearfulness, slow speech, withdrawn posturing.

The Diagnostic Statement also includes items that may or may not be relevant to childhood depressive syndromes: overall rating of anxiety, hostility, and the presence or absence of a number of other specific symptoms—namely, hallucination, delusion, obsession, compulsion, phobia, paranoid ideation, excessive withdrawal, excessive sociability, hyperactivity, and evident impairment in mental functions.

Step 3. Our clinical experience with the children indicated that it was difficult to obtain information on whether the symptoms represented *change* in functioning. Since the children seemed to have marginal comprehension of time perspectives, we developed a parents' questionnaire.

The parents' questionnaire asks whether the child's behavior has *changed* in the specific areas tapped by the items. The questionnaire consists of 25 items, 20 of which specifically relate to depressive symptoms covered in the BDI, phrased in terms of observable behavioral features. Items 21 to 25 tap other behavioral changes that might or might not be associated with childhood depression: increased nervousness, increased demandingness, increased anger, increased dependence, and increased resistance to participate in household activities. Since our pilot interviews with the children also indicated the potential importance of fulfilling parents' expectations, we included eight items in that area.

After we validate the CDI against clinical ratings and aspects of the parents' questionnaire, we plan to work with teachers' ratings as well as levels of actual school performance.

Future Goals

Future steps involve establishing the prevalence and specific characteristics of depressive symptomatology among psychiatric and normal childhood populations. Moreover, eventual investigations on the onset and development of childhood depressive syndromes may be undertaken as a longitudinal study.

The syndrome's psychological characteristics as well as its relationship to specific precipitating factors are additional areas that should be investigated. Such studies together with biological and empirical investigation will eventually contribute to a total understanding of childhood depressive syndromes.

INVESTIGATIONS OF CHILDHOOD DEPRESSION FROM THEORETICAL POINTS OF VIEW

As we already indicated above, we feel that standardized description and measurement of a phenomenon is a necessary first step for bringing order into a confusing field. However, others might take the position that it may be equally feasible to start with existing theories of depression and see if they can illuminate the psychology of childhood depressive disorders. Thus, we briefly summarize and evaluate three types of theories of depression. Our evaluation is focused on whether the theory lends itself to the derivation of hypotheses that can be *operationally* tested and verified.

Psychoanalytic Theory of Depression

Schools of psychoanalytic thought are rather diverse, with varying emphases. For the sake of brevity, we will consider only the original classic psychoanalytic position on depression, which was articulated in its most mature form by Sandor Rado (Gaylin, 1968). Since Rado's 1928 paper built on and clarified points raised by Abraham (1968) and Freud (1968), a brief summary of the latter two is in order.

Abraham initially pointed out the difference between grief and melancholia. Grief, a normal reaction to loss of a love object, differs from melancholia in that the melancholic essentially harbors a great deal of anger and hostility toward the love object. Thus, Abraham's basic position is: (1) the essential problem of the depressed individual derives "from an attitude of the libido in which hatred predominates," and (2) the depressed person suppresses these hostile impulses and experiences them in a changed form, as in the formula "people do not love me, they hate me . . . because of my inborn defects."

Freud (1968) amplified these points and noted that in addition to actual object loss, the loss may be imagined or an unconscious perception. Thus, Freud stated his preconditions for melancholia as follows: (1) loss of a love object, (2) ambivalence toward the lost love object, and (3) regression of libido into the ego. Like Abraham, Freud also stated that in mourning one does *not* see "the disturbance of self-regard" evident in melancholia. The melancholic, according to Freud, is one who has essentially "lost his self-respect."

Freud also clearly called attention to the role of identification (introjection) in depressive phenomena. Upon object-loss, libido is withdrawn into the ego. The withdrawn libido is then used by the ego to identify with the lost object.

Thus, the melancholic regresses from narcissistic object-choice to narcissism and turns his sadism and hate on himself.

Sandor Rado clearly acknowledged the above points and proceeded to delineate the role of the superego in depression. "Fall in the self-esteem and self-satisfaction" are the features that Rado considered most striking in depressive conditions. Moreover, he pointed out that the characteristics that predispose one to depression are intense cravings for narcissistic identification with associated narcissistic intolerance. Thus, such people are *dependent* on love objects for maintaining self-esteem. Even to "trivial offenses and disappointments," they "immediately react with a fall in their self-esteem."

It then follows that such dependent persons react to the threat of withdrawal of love with "embittered vehemence to aggression." However, having withdrawn interest from the object, they withdraw in a narcissistic manner "to the inner world" of their "own mind" and instead of seeking and begging the love of the object, they try to secure that of their own superego.

Developmentally, these processes presume a child of narcissistic disposition whose self-esteem was dependent on the love of his parents. During the time he learned to identify with the parents, he unconsciously discovered that he could punish himself in his own mind and thereby reproduce anticipated punishments. In doing so, he unconsciously wished to win love. In the depressed adult, then, the superego is the instrument of punishment (replacing the parent). The punishment (self-bereavement) is endured by the ego because of its original childhood experience that atonement, through punishment, is the way to win love. Thus, Rado, in his 1928 paper, brings to the forefront two central points: (1) the self-love of depression-prone individuals, and (2) the rage and guilt inherent in depression.

The joint Abraham–Freud–Rado classic psychoanalytic position is a rather complex one that implicates numerous emotions, developmental stages, and psychodynamics in depression: love and hatred, oral-sadistic and oedipal stages, narcissism, identification, introjection, as well as repression and ambivalence, not to mention the basic processes of cathexes and decathexes.

Implications of the Theory for the Psychology of Childhood Depression

Even psychoanalytically oriented authors have feverishly debated whether or not depression can exist among children according to the orthodox analytic formulations. For instance, some authors have indicated that the mechanisms of depression, as outlined, postulate not only a fairly differentiated and strong ego, but also a strong and functioning superego.

To us, it also appears that in the early writings some components of depression tended to be interpreted as regressive phenomena. Consequently, it seems that certain stages of psychosexual and ego development must be completed before a child can show full clinical depression. Although in their original writings Abraham, Freud, and Rado do talk about certain early childhood experiences as necessary for the subsequent development of depression, they do not imply that those experiences signify depression in themselves in the childhood stage in which they occur.

However, our major criticism of the utility of psychoanalytic theory to illuminate psychological aspects of childhood depression lies in a different domain. We have suggested before that a viable theory should lend itself to testable hypotheses. Working hypotheses should define and elucidate new phenomena and lend themselves to empirical verification. In spite of the substantial impact of psychoanalytic theory on the understanding of psychopathology, its tenets have been traditionally and notoriously difficult to submit to empirical investigation. For example, how can you empirically define, quantify, and verify the notion of repressed hostility? Unless future investigators find a way to provide an empirical test of psychoanalytic theories, their contribution to a psychological understanding of childhood depression (as we defined it) remains in doubt.

Learning and Behavioral Theories of Depression

Recently, behaviorally oriented writers have also presented their approach to the concept of depression. From the learning/behaviorist point of view, depression is seen essentially as a function of inadequate or insufficient positive reinforcers, the nature of which might reside in loss of the person who provides reinforcement, lack of the individual's own social skill in making reinforcers available to himself, or role status changes with concomitantly reduced positive reinforcement (Ferster, 1965; Lazarus, 1968; Burgess, 1969; Ullman and Krasner, 1969).

A recent paper by Ferster (1973) is worthy of note because it probably represents a current learning point of view about depression. Ferster begins by summarizing in "learning theory words" the most obvious characteristics of depressed persons, namely: loss of certain kinds of activity, coupled with an increase in avoidance and escape activity such as complaints, crying, and irritability, as well as a noticeable latency in responding. In other words, behavior previously associated with positive reinforcement occurs considerably less frequently, while "aversively motivated behavior," such as requests for help or complaints, increases in frequency. Ferster notes that the aversively motivated behavior either may be "prepotent over," and thus preventive of positively reinforced behavior, or may be a consequence of absence or sudden reduction of positively reinforced behavior.

According to Ferster, depression is often produced within therapy groups by a person's inability to deal with, avoid, or escape from aversive social consequences. Presumably that observation suggests that some depressions may be related to a flaw within the individual's own behavior repertoire.

What behavior processes contribute to or reduce the frequency of positively reinforced behavior? Ferster's answer is that since behavior is the product of

various psychological processes, and since the reduction of positively reinforced behavior is characteristic of various categories of depressed people, we
cannot expect one single underlying causal process.

Ferster considers the dependent variable (frequency of emitted behavior) as
a phenotype that can be caused by many environmental conditions, or geno-
types. Thus, he notes that we cannot yet identify *how* one's "physical and
social environment" provides the conditions for reduction of frequency of
certain emitted behavior.

Ferster then uses clinical descriptions to show how the depressed patient's
behaviors are: (1) not appropriate to changing circumstances in the environment and (2) characterized by lack of normal exploration of the environment
likely to lead to an extended behavior repertoire.

Developmentally, he notes factors that might block the continued enfolding
of a complex and cumulative behavior repertoire. For example, a hiatus in
development caused by inconsistent reinforcement periods or disruptions of
such periods is likely to have negative consequences. He also notes that the
schedule of reinforcement under which behaviors develop will determine their
eventual frequency (e.g., frequently reinforced behaviors will weaken under
intermittent schedules). He especially implicates changes in the environment
(role changes, relationship changes) that require new behavior repertoires as
having an important role in depression.

Taking account of Beck's (1967) clinical observations, Ferster then concludes by stating that a functional analysis of depression can easily take into
account the patient's self-evaluations. He proposes that such a behavioral
analysis would stress the functional relationship of self-evaluative statements
to the person the patient talks to, or to whom he is complaining about himself.

Implications of the Theory for the Psychology of Depression in Childhood

In general, behaviorally oriented workers tend not to be interested in
proving or disproving the presence of a behavior or in explaining the behavior's significance in supra-abstract concept.

The functional analysis of depressive behaviors in adults has no negative
implications for depression in childhood. As a matter of fact, analysis in terms
of avoidance behavior or the reduction of positively reinforced responses
makes depressive phenomena feasible in even the youngest child. Clearly, this
approach emphasizes the operational definition and quantification of behavior.

Nevertheless, our position is that learning/behavioral approaches do not
really illuminate psychological aspects of depression. To be succinct, the
learning/behavioral theorist does not start out by describing or defining
depression. He takes clinicians' designations or descriptions of what constitutes a depressive syndrome and essentially proceeds to observe and define
the observable aspects of people's behavior so classified.

A Cognitive Theory of Depression

Beck's (e.g., 1967,1970,1973,1974*a,b*) theory of depression emphasizes the role of cognitive factors. Beck essentially starts with two basic assumptions: (1) depression is a syndrome or a collection of symptoms, and (2) the diagnosis of depression is dependent on a *change* in the psychobiological systems of the individual.

In contrast to many historic and popular views, Beck's thesis is that "the affective response is determined by the way an individual structures his experience" (Beck, 1967). In the depressed individual, cognition is structured in negative terms, which most often represent faulty and distorted ways of viewing events. Beck assigns a central role to the "cognitive triad" in depression: namely, pervasive negative attitudes that the depressed individual has toward himself, toward the outside world, and toward his future.

1. *The view of self.* The depressed patient's cognitive schemas that relate to self-assessment consist of seeing himself as deficient, inadequate, or unworthy. He often attributes his unpleasant feelings and experiences to some kind of a physical, mental, or moral defect within himself. He then considers himself worthless because of his presumed defect and "rejects" himself.

2. *The view of the world.* The depressed person tends to see his world as making exorbitant demands on him and as presenting obstacles that cannot be surmounted. He interprets his interactions with his environment in terms of defeat and failure, deprivation, or disparagement.

3. *The view of the future.* The depressed person's negative cognitive patterns that relate to the future become evident in his view that his current difficulties or suffering will continue indefinitely. Thus, he anticipates unremitting hardship, continued frustration, and never-ending deprivation. Such schemas essentially amount to a pervasive hopeless attitude.

According to Beck, the hallmark of the negative cognitive triad is that the negative evaluations are unrealistic, distorted, and illogical ways of thinking that do not correspond to reality. The distorted and illogical ways of thinking are manifested in the depressed person's tendencies to make extravagant use of the following processes: exaggerating or misinterpreting events; making extreme, absolute judgments in certain situations; overgeneralizing from a single incident; focusing on one particular detail out of context and ignoring the more salient features of a situation; drawing inferences in the absence of or even contrary to evidence; and extracting personally relevant meanings from unpleasant situations.

Moreover, the content of the negative thought patterns tends to revolve around themes of loss and deprivation. As Beck has noted, the word "loser" pretty much captures the flavor of the depressive's appraisal of himself, his experience, and his future. In cases of actual losses, the depressive individual tends to exaggerate the loss, misinterpret it, or attach overgeneralized or extravagant meaning to it. Furthermore, the depressed individual often dwells on what may be called "hypothetical" losses and "pseudo" losses.

According to Beck, most of the depressive symptoms (e.g., motivational, mood, and behavior changes) seem to result from the depressed person's primarily negative and distorted ways of thinking. Thus, if an individual's conceptualization of himself or of a situation has an unpleasant content, he will experience a corresponding unpleasant affective response. Beck also traces symptoms such as indecisiveness, paralysis of the will, avoidance wishes, suicidal wishes, and increased dependency to the patient's negative view of himself, of his world, and of his future.

For example, the cognitive theory of depression considers the depressed person's negative view of the self as a primary determinant of the self-blame commonly observed in such individuals. One of the prominent schemas in depressed individuals is that somehow they are "deficient." Consequently, it makes sense that they consider themselves blameworthy, feel remorse, and remain essentially passive in the face of adversity and even deprivation.

Although the etiological-developmental aspects of this theory have not yet been worked out in detail, Beck has speculated that certain unfavorable life situations such as the loss of a parent, chronic rejection by peers, or insidious stresses may sensitize an individual to become "depression prone." The earlier unfavorable experiences may predispose the individual to overreact to analogous conditions in later life. Beck has also speculated that individuals who, even as children, tended to set up rigid and perfectionistic goals for themselves may also be especially "depression prone." When such individuals eventually confront disappointments in life, their universe literally collapses. However, it must be kept in mind that "the specific stresses responsible for adult depressions impinge on the individual's specific vulnerability" (Beck, 1974b).

Implications of the Theory for the Psychology of Childhood Depression

Critics of the cognitive model of depression (e.g., Izard, 1972) have pointed out a number of weak points: (1) the theory essentially ignores the motivational properties of emotion; (2) it has difficulty accounting for the overt physiological and vegetative symptoms of depression; and (3) the actual etiology of persistently negative views of the self, the world, and the future is obscure.

However, Beck himself (1967) has admitted the possibility and the feasibility that the depressive syndrome might consist of a circular feedback model in which cognition feeds into affect and so forth. He has also acknowledged that points 2 and 3 are yet to be worked out. Even in view of some of the theory's weaknesses, it has implications for illuminating the psychology of childhood depression. It is immensely practical and useful because the cognitive conceptualization of depression can be relatively easily operationalized and lends itself to empirical verification.

Anyone wishing to start from this theoretical point of view and attempt to undertake empirical analyses of the psychology of childhood depression will find numerous examples in our work with adults (e.g., Loeb, Feshbach, Beck, and Wolf, 1964; Beck, 1967; Loeb, Beck, Diggory, and Tuthill, 1967; Loeb, Beck, and Diggory, 1971). For example, negative expectations or self-view may be operationally defined in terms of a subject's verbally stated expectations of success or failure in an experimental task. Since outcome on a task can be experimentally manipulated, it is easy to prearrange success or failure experiences. The cognitive theory predicts that depressed patients will exaggerate and overgeneralize. Thus, a failure experience could be expected to produce more pervasive negative expectations with respect to subsequent task performance.

Tasks such as card sorting, picture sorting, or the like lend themselves to easy determination of the actual level of performance. Such measures can be compared to depressed subjects' estimates or evaluations and can be compared with those of normals to determine the degree of cognitive distortion of current experience. The thesis that depression involves a disorder of thinking can also be empirically tested along the lines described by Braff and Beck (1974).

In our work with adults, we have developed an instrument that quantifies the construct of hopelessness (Beck, Weissman, Lester, and Trexler, 1974). A similarly constructed instrument that is appropriate to children may be employed to examine the effect of positive experimental play or interactional experiences.

A potentially important aspect of this theory is that it may be integrated with theories of cognitive development, such as Piaget's. According to Piaget's theories of cognitive and language development, within the late preoperational and the full concrete operational stages (roughly from ages 6 or 7 to 11), a child is capable of defining properties and understanding certain relations. Moreover, he becomes capable of kinetic and transformational imagery as well as of using language as a vehicle of communication (Ginsburg and Opper, 1969).

This theory, together with the cognitive theory of depression, may be of value in presenting an integrated approach toward understanding the psychology of childhood depression, as well as outlining some of its unique properties.

SUMMARY

Description of a phenomenon and its reliable assessment are necessary first steps in order to build up a scientific body of knowledge. In order to bring clarity into the area of childhood depression, our strategy is to proceed from the known to the unknown. It is known that depressive syndromes can be delineated and measured among adults. The available literature indicates that a similar discriminable set of behaviors may exist among children. The accurate description and assessment of this phenomenon is necessary for subsequent inquiry into the nosology, etiology, correlates, and treatment of childhood depressive disorders.

We have described our pilot studies of the description and systematic assessment of depressive symptoms among children and discussed their implications. We also outlined future steps necessary to bring about a solid clinical and theoretical understanding of childhood depressive syndromes. We pointed out the assets and shortcomings of some currently existing theories in the empirical study of childhood depression.

REFERENCES

Abraham, K. Notes on the psychoanalytical investigation and treatment of manic-depressive insanity and allied conditions. In W. Gaylin (ed.): *The Meaning of Despair*. New York, Science House, pp. 26–49, 1968.

Albert, N. *Evidence of Depression in an Early Adolescent School Population*. Unpublished manuscript, Villanova, Pennsylvania, 1973.

Albert, N., and Beck, A. T. Incidence of depression in early adolescence: A preliminary study. *J. Youth Adolescence*, 4:301–307, 1975.

Arajärvi, T., and Huttunen, M. Encopresis and enuresis as symptoms of depression. In A. L. Annell (ed.): *Depressive States in Childhood and Adolescence*. Stockholm, Almqvist and Wiksell, 212–217, 1972.

Bakwin, H. Depression—a mood disorder in children and adolescents. *Md. State Med. J.*, 55–61, 1972.

Beck, A. T. *Depression: Clinical, Experimental and Theoretical Aspects*. New York, Harper & Row, 1967.

Beck, A. T. The core problem in depression: The cognitive triad. In J. H. Masserman (ed.): *Depression: Theories and Therapies*. New York, Grune & Stratton, 1970.

Beck, A. T. Measuring depression: The depression inventory. In T. A. Williams, M. M. Katz, and J. A. Shield (eds.): *Recent Advances in the Psychobiology of the Depressive Illnesses*. Washington, Government Printing Office, 299–302, 1972.

Beck, A. T. *The Diagnosis and Management of Depression*. Philadelphia, University of Pennsylvania Press, 1973.

Beck, A. T. Depressive neurosis. In S. Arieti (ed.): *American Handbook of Psychiatry, Vol. III*, Ed. 2. New York, Basic Books, pp. 61–90, 1974a.

Beck, A. T. The development of depression: A cognitive model. In R. Friedman and M. Katz (eds.): *Psychology of Depression: Contemporary Theory and Research*. Washington, D.C., Winston-Wiley, pp. 3–27, 1974b.

Beck, A. T., and Beamesderfer, A. Assessment of depression: The depression inventory. In P. Pichot (Ed.): *Psychological measurements in psychopharmacology, Mod. Probl. Pharmacopsychiatry*, Vol. 7, 151–169, Basel, Karger, 1974.

Beck, A. T., and Beck, R. W. Screening depressed patients in family practice: A rapid technic. *Postgrad. Med.*, 52:81–85, 1972.

Beck, A. T., Rial, W., and Rickels, K. Short form of depression inventory: Cross validation. *Psychol. Rep.*, 34:1184–1186, 1974.

Beck, A. T., Weissman, A., Lester, D., and Trexler, L.: The measurement of pessimism: The hopelessness scale. *J. Consult. Clin. Psychol.*, 42:861–865, 1974.

Braff, D. L., and Beck, A. T. Thinking disorder in depression. *Arch. Gen. Psychiatry*, 31:456–459, 1974.

Burgess, E. P. The modification of depressive behaviors. In R. Rubin and C. Franks (eds.): *Advances in Behavior Therapy*. New York, Academic Press, pp. 193–199, 1969.

Connell, H. M. Depression in childhood. *Child Psychiatry Hum. Dev.*, 4:71–85, 1972.

Cytryn, L., and McKnew, D. H. Factors influencing the changing clinical expression of the depressive process in children. *Am. J. Psychiatry*, 131:879–881, 1974.

Ferster, C. B. Classification of behavioral pathology. In L. Krasner and L. P. Ullman (eds.): *Research in Behavior Modification*. New York, Holt, Rinehart and Winston, pp. 6–26, 1965.

Ferster, C. B. A functional analysis of depression. *Am. Psychol.*, 28:857–869, 1973.

Freud, S. Mourning and melancholia. In W. Gaylin (ed.): *The Meaning of Despair*. New York, Science House, pp. 50–69, 1968.

Frommer, E. Depressive illness in childhood. *Br. J. Psychiatry*, 2:117–123, 1968.

Gaylin, W. (ed.): *The Meaning of Despair*. New York, Science House, 1968.

Ginsburg, H., and Opper, S. *Piaget's Theory of Intellectual Development*. Englewood Cliffs, N.J., Prentice-Hall, 1969.

Glaser, K. Masked depression in children and adolescents. *Annu. Prog. Child Psychiatry Child Dev.*, 1:345–355, 1968.

Izard, C. E. *Patterns of Emotions*. New York, Academic Press, 1972.

Krakowski, A. J. Depressive reactions of childhood and adolescence. *Psychosomatics*, 11:429–433, 1970.

Kuhn, V., and Kuhn, R. Drug therapy for depression in children. Indications and methods. In A. L. Annell (ed.): *Depressive States in Childhood and Adolescence*. Stockholm, Almqvist and Wiksell, pp. 455–459, 1972.

Lazarus, A. Learning theory and the treatment of depression. *Behav. Res. Ther.*, 6:83–89, 1968.

Ling, W., Oftedal, G., and Weinberg, W. Depressive illness in childhood presenting as severe headache. *Am. J. Dis. Child.*, 120:122–124, 1970.

Loeb, A., Beck, A. T., and Diggory, J. Differential effects of success and failure on depressed and nondepressed patients. *J. Nerv. Ment. Dis.*, 152:106–114, 1971.

Loeb, A., Beck, A. T., Diggory, J. C., and Tuthill, R. Expectancy, level of aspiration, performance, and self-evaluation in depression. *Proceedings of the 75th Annual Convention of the American Psychological Association, Vol. 2*, 193–194, 1967.

Loeb, A., Feshbach, S., Beck, A. T., and Wolf, A.: Some effect of reward upon the social perception and motivation of psychiatric patients varying in depression. *J. Abnorm. Soc. Psychol.*, 68:609–616, 1964.

Malmquist, C. P. Depressive phenomena in children. In B. B. Wolman (ed.): *Manual of Child Psychopathology*. New York, McGraw-Hill, pp. 497–540, 1972.

McConville, B. J., Boag, L. C., and Purohit, A. P. Three types of childhood depression. *Can. Psychiat. Assoc. J.*, 18:133–138, 1973.

Poznanski, E., and Zrull, J. P. Childhood depression: Clinical characteristics of overtly depressed children. *Arch. Gen. Psychiatry*, 23:8–15, 1970.

Rado, S. Psychodynamics of depression from the etiologic point of view. In W. Gaylin (ed.): *The Meaning of Despair*. New York, Science House, pp. 96–107, 1968.

Renshaw, D. C. Suicide and depression in children. *J. School Health*, 44:487–489, 1974.

Toolan, J. M. Depression in children and adolescents. *Am. J. Orthopsychiatry*, 32:404–414, 1962.

Ullman, L. P., and Krasner, L. *A Psychological Approach to Abnormal Behavior*. Englewood Cliffs, N.J., Prentice-Hall, 1969.

Vranješević, D., Radiojičić, B., Bumbaširević, S., and Todorivić, S. Depressive manifestations in children with intracranial tumors. In A. L. Annell (ed.): *Depressive States in Childhood and Adolescence*. Stockholm, Almqvist and Wiksell, pp. 201–206, 1972.

Weinberg, W. A., Rutman, J., Sullivan, L., Penick, E. C., and Dietz, S. G. Depression in children referred to an educational diagnostic center: Diagnosis and treatment. *J. Pediatr.*, 83:1065–1072, 1973.

Discussion of the Chapter by Drs. Kovacs and Beck:
An Empirical-Clinical Approach Toward a Definition of Childhood

Anthony Nowels

Departments of Child Psychiatry and Psychiatry, University of Miami School of Medicine, Miami, Florida 33124

I felt slightly out of place reviewing "An Empirical-Clinical Approach Toward a Definition of Childhood Depression" because my work has been primarily with adolescents. On the other hand, I felt that I should advocate that adolescents be included since everyone else seems to ignore the adolescent age group. We have worked extensively with depressed adolescents, and if I had any one recommendation to start with, it would be to consider the adolescent depressive as having his or her own special problems and treatment needs.

The chapter of Drs. Kovacs and Beck is a delight. I'm excited to see this kind of empirical research begun in the area of childhood and adolescence. Since I do not have the time to review the chapter the way I would like, I have the freedom to give some of my own ideas and thoughts along the way.

First, Drs. Kovacs and Beck had the courage to proceed in the face of widespread disagreement and confusion within the field and say, "We are going to take a stand in a particular area and begin to look at some hard data and ignore a lot of other things." This, even though others may say, "Well you haven't taken this or that into account," or "There is a long list of things to be added after that," etc. They have not allowed the confusion and the morass of unknowns to keep them from getting to work. They appear to assume that we are all starting from a particular point where we can agree that: depression does exist, it can be measured, it exists in children, and it can exist in any child. I would add that it probably exists much more commonly than we realize and that additional research in this area is necessary.

At the 100th meeting of the National Mental Health Advisory Council, there was some exciting talk about adult work by Drs. Daniel Freeman and William Bunney. Adult work in the area of depression isn't really as clear or concise as people might imagine. Drs. Kovacs and Beck made several references to the adult depression work in their chapter, which also indicates the large amount of work that needs to be done. Additional research in children and adolescents is even more needed.

Their chapter points out the difficulty we all have in defining depression, including all the different ways we use the term: as a symptom, as an illness, as some kind of central feeling state or peripheral physiology, or even as a normal feeling. The biggest problem we have had is limiting the term, and this is particularly true for "masked depressions," an idea I would like to promote because my feeling is quite different from Dr. Beck's in this regard. I believe masked depression is a useful concept. However, one can fill, as we did, a whole adolescent ward with depressives if the meaning of the terms masked depressions or depressive equivalents is not limited. I hope that as we try to define depression, we include the notion that we have to *limit* our concepts as well. Being too inclusive restricts the value of the concept.

Childhood and adolescent depression encompasses a broad range of behaviors. Someone mentioned the juvenile justice system, and certainly it has been our impression as well that enormous numbers of children in various areas of our society display all kinds of behaviors that people either like or dislike that may be related to depression. The question of where normalcy ends and pathology begins is just such a dilemma and one we will have to address eventually.

One other subject Dr. Kovacs alluded to that I think needs even more emphasis is childhood development. We are lumping together toddlers, school-age children, preadolescents, and adolescents. This covers a multitude of areas, and I think more attention needs to be given to that. This is not to say that development stops with adulthood, but most people feel that children change more quickly than adults and that in children some of the changes are more dramatic. Our experience, for example, with the Beck Depression Inventory (BDI) in adolescents has been that, depending on where they are developmentally (and I don't mean age-wise so much as cognitively), the inability to respond meaningfully to the questions varies widely. A group of younger adolescents may reject items or laugh at the questions, finding them totally alien to their way of looking at the world, whereas an older group may deal with them much more successfully. So I think we must consider where kids are developmentally and how they will look at the questions.

The National Institute of Mental Health Collaborative Depression Study Group, of course, is studying an issue that Drs. Kovacs and Beck wanted to avoid—namely, nosology and classification. I think we will have to consider this eventually. If we have a whole legacy of adult work in depression, then I feel comfortable that we can begin extrapolating from that to childhood. Nature does not develop things with extreme discontinuity. The notion that childhood depression is something totally alien, separate, and discontinuous from adult depression is not something that one teleologically likes to think about. So I support taking the "knowns" of the adult world and extrapolating backward. It may be very fruitful, but it is only a beginning.

Another issue has to do with the concept of *time,* which is quite different for children and adults. When one is applying a self-report instrument, a child's idea of what he or she is talking about with respect to time has to be taken into account. Especially for younger children, the preceding 10 min may be the most important part of their lives, and the importance of that and its significance in terms of defining an illness need more work.

Also with respect to time, what happens to these depressed children over long periods? We must develop longitudinal studies. For example, our group certainly sees a number of adolescents who have been diagnosed as having depression—some are depressed kids who have many psychotic features early in adolescence. What happens when they become adults? Do they retain those psychotic features or do they become adult depressives? I don't know the answer. All the issues relating to genetic, environmental, and particularly biological questions have to be raised and resolved from that point.

The magnitude of those tasks is enormous. Confusion tends to exhaust one, but Dr. Kovacs has been able to go beyond that and take a stand. I think his approach is basically sound. It is especially important to operationalize these concepts, and it is exciting that this group has been able to start. Yet it is also important to emphasize that we are dealing with a subgroup of depressions. Dr. Kovacs' group has already rejected a large number of depressive equivalents. I suspect that the group they picked represents a "more self-aware" subgroup, and I think that needs to be said at the start.

The review of the literature was good. It pointed out what has been mentioned in several articles recently, i.e., that there really have not been the kinds of adequately controlled studies that need to be done in children, where one can take the data and begin to operationalize the concepts mentioned. Many papers on children and adolescents do not have the kinds of controls and methods required if the study is to include all the important concepts. Do we even know if we've asked all the right questions? Obviously, we do not, but with what Dr. Kovacs has outlined, I think we can ask better questions.

The parents' questionnaire is quite important, although we might begin to develop questionnaires for "significant others," including parents, teachers, etc. We need more family and other input for hard data and also additional family validation of the actual material that the children are asked to fill out. This also relates, in part, to the question about the children's concept of time. Some validation of how children use time could come from parents' and teachers' reports as well. Also, I am not sure that children, and this was my experience with adolescents, have quite the same judgment about notions of severity as adults do. Gerald Klerman and others have written that severely depressed patients are less able to make accurate judgments about the severity of their illness than patients less severely depressed. I think that may also apply to children.

We must also consider moving away from simple self-report. We need physicians' ratings, school input, and with adolescents perhaps peer input. With our own group of 13- to 17-year-olds, we ask the adolescents on our service to rate each other. We use the word depression without defining it for them. We also ask them to rate anger, overall functioning, and group interaction. I'm not always sure what to do with these ratings, and I don't know their validity or reliability, but I think they are interesting to think about with respect to older children and adolescents.

The extreme depressive response of the normal 7th and 8th graders to me was striking. I didn't know what to do with that.

I had to ask myself first if there is that much depression or some equivalent feeling in the normal group. I'd love to have had some additional clinical data with some of those kids just to see what they were doing. In part there may be that much depression. According to some conservative estimates, children have a very high incidence of depression or depressive equivalents. Teacher estimates are at least as high as 10 or 15%; clinical adult studies have been as high as 16%. But other problems may be distorting those items. First, they may reflect child development, e.g., a 7- or 8-year-old has some age-appropriate fears about mastering skills or confidence and questions his self-esteem. Thus, normal developmental problems or fears rather than true depression may be detected.

The 7th or 8th graders are honest when they answer questions about suicide. They might answer in a way that doesn't take into account any interpretation of what you are going to do with that question, in the same way that an adult would.

There is the issue of communication. I was a little puzzled by what Dr. Kovacs said about children not using language for communication until age 7. I think it probably starts at approximately 6 months. We certainly took into account some of what was said in terms of our use of the BDI with adolescents because I think it must be phrased carefully whether they are performing formal operations and are comfortable with symbolic thinking or whether they are doing concrete operations and are not comfortable with that. We can, I believe, use language and verbal communication with children earlier than age 7.

I agree with Drs. Kovacs and Beck that we need a much better definition of masked depression or depressive equivalents. In Miami we have tended to start with a puristic definition. In a group of adolescents who were referred we feel depression is a major portion of what is going on, yet they were not diagnosed by good clinicians on the outside as having depression. Maybe that just means we should retrain people in diagnosis and not come up with a concept of masked depression. However, I feel there are biological equivalents going on centrally, that one has in the absence of either cognitive or symptomatic issues that would, for example, respond to antidepressant medication, and therefore would be useful in terms of treatment of masked depression. I think we must consider central nervous system biochemistry versus peripheral symptomatology.

In summary, I think Drs. Kovacs and Beck made a marvelous start, and I'm looking forward to the data on pathological or depressed kids. I want to support what Dr. McKinney said about training and research leading to the major goals. We must describe and define depression, and we have to get into issues of classification and nosology and biology at some point. I would like to see more high-risk designs, which we are working with now and which may give us valuable information. I think this group should work toward a better epidemiology data base from which to begin to make judgments and from which to develop hypotheses. I also think the self-report must be supplemented by other kinds of assessment instruments, especially those including the family. Finally, I am looking forward to using the Childhood Depression Inventory (CDI).

Depression in Childhood: Diagnosis, Treatment, and Conceptual Models, edited by J. G. Schulterbrandt and A. Raskin. Raven Press, New York, 1977.

Childhood Depression: A Clinical and Behavioral Perspective

Carl P. Malmquist

Law School and Department of Criminal Justice, University of Minnesota, Minneapolis, Minnesota 55455

QUESTIONS THAT NEED ASKING

The approach I am going to use is that of raising questions about the nature of childhood depressions. I believe these questions need asking if we are to progress beyond our present level of understanding. Since simple questions are usually the best, let us begin with one: What is a childhood depression? Most of this chapter is devoted to elaboration of this question. To begin with a nosological aside, no category of childhood depression is available if we limit ourselves to the *Diagnostic Manual* (1968) of the American Psychiatric Association. Why is no such diagnosis included in the section on "Behavior Disorders of Childhood and Adolescence"? Rather, we find reactions of children listed, such as overactivity, inattentiveness, overaggressiveness, shyness, a feeling of rejection, timidity, and group delinquency. Although we might insert a depressed child into one of the diagnostic categorizations used with adults, this does not account for the omission. Various hypotheses and explanations to account for this deficit could be offered, and those of us with a historical curiosity about the changing views of how we approach childhood psychopathology could contribute a paper devoted to this topic alone.

One of the greatest omissions in most approaches to childhood depressions is the lack of a developmental perspective. This is even more striking than mutual omissions between those seeking organic correlates and those looking for psychodynamic contributory factors. This is where I think the contributions of child psychiatrists should be maximal. Their natural interest in child development, aided by direct clinical work with children, should lend insights. It is acceptable for a debate, even among skilled clinicians, as to when true neurotic conflict exists so that a depressive neurosis is present, but there would be little debate about depressive affect as a developmental phenomenon which can be experienced quite early in life. Such affect is experienced in response to many situations and in different quantities. All of these responses are not psychopathological, e.g., the need to mourn which is a necessary part of grieving. This can occur in response to specific losses but also in the form of coming to terms with changes taking place within the child and his environment. Sad affect in a child, like more general moods, does not mean the child is clinically depressed.

What if we progress a step further where we recognize a conscious conflict exists? An infant deprived of "good mothering" is thus observed to become apathetic, sleep poorly, eat fitfully if at all, and in time fail to thrive. The response to deprivation, or the misinterpretation of it, seems related to this set of reactive symptoms. Similarly, a depressed parent may complain about his latency-age child's performance in school having fallen off and report that the child does not appear interested in anything anymore and seems to lack vitality. Such an example again reflects depressive affect, but not at the level where it is a fixed personality pattern or is entwined with unconscious meanings to a degree sufficient for a neurosis.

Given these types of situations, it is also possible that over sufficient time, certain mood instabilities gain prominence. At that point they are not removed when the precipitating events are gone. If we prolong the period of insufficient caretaking, reversibility in the child becomes more difficult. We become aware of the vista of theoretical problems from the diverse orientations of people interested in developmental aspects of depression. As one example, consider the studies dealing with deprived animals, especially monkeys. I find these studies fascinating and I envy the type of rigorousness they can employ, particularly since this is rarely available to the clinician. To what extent are we permitted to extend their findings to the problem of how children react with depressive affect? Monkeys reared in isolation later show retarded and deviant social behavior in comparison to other monkeys, and the former are called "depressed." A conclusion is made that reactive symptoms, or even developmental deviations, are not immutable since these depressed monkeys can be "cured" by placing them with younger female monkeys for a 26-week period (Suomi and Harlow, 1972). In addition to the reversibility of such depressions, or rather reactive states, we must also question the ongoing development of an organism in a maturational sense when confronted with environmental adversities.

A diversity of specific questions can be raised about childhood depressions. For brevity, they will be asked initially without any accompanying discussion. Suggestive answers to some of these questions appear throughout this chapter.

1. What is the actual incidence of different types of depressions in childhood? How often do reactive depressive disturbances occur in children in contrast to other types of reactive manifestations?

2. When do we begin to see developmental deviations ensuing therefrom? Or, what variety of developmental problems related to depression are possible?

3. When do we begin to see actual depressive neuroses in children? What is the nature of the debate about this issue in both theoretical and empirical terms?

4. What types of family transitional states are most likely to give rise to childhood depressions? It is presumptuous to say that these must be restricted to one type of event, such as death or divorce of a parent. Many other interpersonal phenomena occur as well as variations in how a child adapts to situations.

5. What intrapsychic events are most related to a depressive diathesis? We talk of loss, but what makes for the different sensitivities to loss in different children? The variables of a child's ego strength cannot be ignored.

6. Since children, or their parents, rarely come complaining that the child is depressed, in contrast to the mode of presentation in adults, we need clarification on a descriptive level of the nature of childhood depression. In that manner, by recording and classifying symptomatology, we will begin to obtain a more valid base line regarding the incidence of disturbances in this area.

7. The next step is to have longitudinal studies dealing with the outcome of childhood depressive phenomena. At this point, apart from retrospective impressions based on work with adults in therapy, we do not know the diverse pathways by direct follow-up from such a group of children. We actually have more knowledge about socially deprived children who are environmentally neglected.

8. Do depressive disorders in children differ in parts of the country and world? This is simply a variation on the impact of different cultural contexts.

9. What kinds of dreams do depressed children have? These could be studied by the manifest content if we were going to quantify, or by clinical significance as in therapy.

10. Finally, discussion about a particular condition, for whatever reason, increases the frequency of its diagnosis. Hence, one clinic reported that when phenothiazines were reported as alleviating schizophrenic symptomatology, the diagnosis of schizophrenia became more frequent; when lithium received more publicity several years later, the diagnosis of affective disorders increased in the same clinic (Baldesserini, 1970). I predict that childhood depressions will increase in popularity over the next decade as a diagnosis.

EARLY STUDIES

Early manifestations of depression are often lumped together within some vague grouping of "infantile depressions." Part of this vagueness is associated with the old problem in comprehending anything connected with depressive phenomena since all or only one of the following may be present: (1) a symptom of sadness present in depressions or with other clinical diagnoses; (2) a mood state; (3) a depressive syndrome with certain signs and symptoms which may then receive a diagnosis. Note that none of these possibilities deals with etiology or the subtypes of diagnoses of depressions.

Reliance on retrospective data from children and adults who manifest some particular part of this spectrum adds to the skepticism about our knowledge of depression. Efforts have been made to extend directly a "deprivation hypothesis" to longitudinal studies of such children. Early reports had the methodological difficulty of dealing with children not only of different ages but also in different settings such as nurseries, foster homes, hospitals, and diverse institutions. Different personnel observed disruptions in the capacity to form consistent human attachments based on an affectional deprivation.

Another line of approach stressed the associated deficits in cognitive-intellectual functioning. Early childhood was seen as the vulnerable contributing period. Some of these approaches were based on clinical work. Others were from work with the mentally or emotionally retarded. Not until later was the animal model for studying depressions introduced with its own set of methodological problems in transferring conclusions to children. Biochemical models came even later, again using animals for behavioral observations or chance consequences, such as reserpine precipitating depressions in humans.

The problems that arise in studying the developmental phenomenon of depressive proneness are similar to those encountered in investigating many areas of biopsychosocial development (Eisenberg, 1971). This work was begun in the 1920s and 1930s. Although we can find fault with many of the early investigators' approaches, before then childhood depressions were either ignored as psychological phenomena or seen as unexplained cachexias. Thus, Levy (1937) reported on an 8-year-old girl who had been in a succession of foster homes and then adopted. The child continued to manifest an incapacity to form attachments described as a lack of emotional responsiveness and as having a "hunger" for affect. In 1943 Goldfarb studied 30 children, ages 34 to 35 months, and concluded that 15 of the children brought up in institutions had IQs 28 points lower than those raised in foster homes since the age of 4 months. Observations on children placed in the Hampstead nursery during the bombing of London in World War II revealed less-serious maternal deprivation repercussions for the older child, but the effects were more serious when occurring at an earlier age (Burlingham and Freud, 1943). Again, it is interesting to call attention to how such clinical observations received confirmatory evidence 30 years later from animal workers who found that traumatic separations of monkeys in infancy predisposed them later to despair reactions on separation, whereas those separated at 3 to 4 years of age exhibited only protest types of responses (Young et al., 1973).

Nevertheless, the question of whether emotional harm is greater from experiences that occur at a younger age remains controversial and unsettled. Clinical impressions based on the greater biological vulnerability of the young organism continue to favor this hypothesis. However, developmentally, the younger organism possesses a greater adaptive capacity, such as being able to accept substitute objects, which can work in its favor. In this early work there is some confusion among emotional deprivation, lack of sufficient maternal care, possible organic cerebral impairment, and the syndrome of infantile depression.

The syndrome of "anaclitic depression," elaborated by Spitz (1946), is actually a deprivation reaction. Pediatricians encountering this condition in children called it "marasmus," but the best they could do was view it as some type of degenerative or dystrophic disease. Spitz recognized that after objective recognition at 6 months, separation led to a grief reaction if the relationship with the maternal object had been previously satisfactory. We now realize that the earliest types of perceptual and attachment behaviors occur from the earliest period of contact with a maternal object. Infants in such situations become sad, weepy, apathetic, and have immobile faces with a distant look. They react slowly to stimuli, exhibit retarded movements, have anorexia and insomnia, and show little of the motility characteristic of infants. The diagnosis of depression was attached since these behaviors appeared similar to those in adults who were depressed. After 3 months of such a separation, a full restoration to emotional capacity was believed rare.

Similar symptoms and signs were observed in children institutionalized as infants and kept separated from their mothers without adequate stimulation and fondling. This had more serious overtones since both mental and physical development lagged, repeated infections were common, and in some cachexia and even death occurred. The clinical picture described as "hospitalism" emerged from its frequent association with children maintained in emotionally sterile institutional settings. A similar clinical picture was seen in infants with gastric fistulas (Engel and Reichsman, 1956; Coddington, 1968). Engel and Reichsman hypothesized a "depression-withdrawal" reaction in their fistulic infant. In the presence of a stranger, inactivity, hypotonia, a sad facial expression, decreased gastric secretion, and finally sleep occurred. Subsequent studies attempted to appraise this work on institutionalized children.

Criticism centered on methodological considerations and questions as to how adequate the physical evaluation procedures employed had been. Infants with nutritional deficiencies may appear indistinguishable from those subject to prolonged institutionalization. Even more striking is the similarity with nonhuman primates in which signs of distress are witnessed similar to the anaclitic depression in human infants (Kaufman and Rosenblum, 1967). Brief separation experiences produce symptoms in rhesus monkey infants similar to those in human infants (Hinde and Spencer-Booth, 1971). Such variables as age at the time of separation, length of separation, and sex of the infant need consideration since different behavioral consequences are associated with these variables (Young et al., 1973). Most impressive are reports from animal work that the effects of experimental work with subhuman mammals last for months or years even in certain brief separations.

In 1951, *Maternal Care and Mental Health* reviewed previous studies and presented new formulations (Bowlby, 1951). There have been subsequent updatings (*Perspective on Human Deprivation,* 1968; Rutter, 1972), yet radically different conclusions have not emerged. There is consistency of certain hypotheses on one hand, and on the other the usual type of refining of hypotheses by criticism of methodology and lack of conceptual clarity. One of the major difficulties in appraising these studies is to separate the impact of "maternal deprivation" as one antecedent relating to the genesis of depression from the syndrome of maternal deprivation *per se,* which appears as a depression. Different kinds of deprivation—psychological, social, cognitive, and organic—must be specified. This need for specificity has been the greatest obstacle in attempts to unravel the effects subsumed under maternal deprivation. Not until specific independent variables are tied up as components of depressive proneness will higher correlations in outcome studies of development be possible.

The critiques have sought to select several of the factors frequently mentioned as related to an outcome of depressive proneness. It was originally felt that prolonged disruptions during the first 3 years of life had a certain impact on the child's personality, such as appearing emotionally withdrawn and isolated. This was seen particularly in children maintained in nurseries and residential settings with "inadequate mothering." This variable is now seen as only one of many. Other family members may have a significnt impact, as may other individuals with whom the children are in contact, especially if these other individuals are conflicted and have depressive problems of their own. In addition, the various types of perceptual and cognizing experiences of a child influence the way he begins to view the world. Early cognitive components emerge related to whether a child thinks of the world as a place where people are happy or as a "vale of tears." Nor can the whole panoply of organic and genetic factors as antecedents toward certain lines of development be ignored (Berger and Passingham, 1973).

In the early writings about maternal deprivation, various outcomes were predicted, including psychosis, neurosis, and delinquency. This type of hypothesizing is so broad as to be unrefuted; endless confirmations occurred but never the crucial observations to refute. A more specific hypothesis asks if a particular type of deprivation has any specific etiologic role for the later emergence of depressive vulnerability. Further, is this manifest then in childhood, adolescence, or adulthood? Even though details are lacking about the specific mechanism governing why some children are fortunate enough to be excluded from later consequences, the hypothesis can be tested. Distinctions are now made between disruption of affectionate relationships which have already been established, and which are more conducive to a depressive outcome, and relationships which have failed to form are then more related to psychopathy.

There has been criticism of the heavy emphasis in maternal deprivation formulations that outcomes are rigidly proscribed in the earliest months of a child's life. There is a tacit assumption that early mother-child relationships inevitably lead to certain outcomes. It is basically a hope that if we knew all the variables, we could predict a depressive or a psychopathic outcome. Such a degree of specificity has not been established. The concept is weighted in the direction of an overemphasis on early infantile experiences leading to an unalterable outcome without sufficient cognizance of other significant variables in the child's life. Wooton (1959) has pointed out that subsequent broader influences in a child's life—such as school associations, vocation, and marriage—are not sufficiently accounted for but can taper and modify early experiences. The inevitability may not be so, nor the irreversibility. Other specific experiences contribute to depressive proneness. Death of a friend, pet, or neighbor contributes as well as that of a parent. Nor is deprivation to be considered literally in terms of losing an attachment to a person since moving to a new neighborhood can elicit similar feelings. Symbolic losses are seen as significant no less frequently than traumatic separations from a loved one.

EARLY PSYCHODYNAMIC FORMULATIONS

Clinical knowledge concerning depressions in adults began within the framework of descriptive psychiatry. Freud and Abraham extended this work by psychoanalytic theorizing, which raised psychological hypotheses about what had occurred during the childhood of the depressed. The earliest formulations saw childhood as significant to the extent that a "trauma" left a child vulnerable to depressive illness. These traumas were viewed primarily as retrospective curiosities. Concepts such as orality, introjection, turning against the self, narcissistic injury, loss of an object, anal-sadism, and ambivalence were introduced as explanatory constructs to account for the development and maintenance of depressed states. In 1911 Abraham emphasized the repression of aggression leading to depression analogous to the postulation of "actual neuroses" being from repression of sexuality leading to anxiety.

The theory of psychosexual stages led to knowledge about fixations and regressions. Introjective processes with their attendant ambivalence, along with regressions to anal-sadistic and oral cannibalistic stages, were the mechanisms postulated intrapsychically. Regression subsequent to loss of a love object was part of the early theorizing (Freud, 1917). Abraham (1924) expanded this to include the mechanism of double introjection. The original love object is introjected as part of the ego-ideal and conscience; it then becomes subject to hostile attacks as well. Developmentally, a crucial step relevant to depressions is the child treating the internalized object as something over which control is exercised. This is similar to the way in which control over other possessions, such as body parts and contents, is perceived. An equation is made between loss of such objects and loss of bodily possessions. The cognitive antithesis is: "losing-destroying" versus "retaining-controlling." Emergence of depressive proneness in a child reveals an emphasis on control and orderliness—the basic obsessional personality seen in the compensated depressive as he matures.

These early formulations about intrapsychic mechanisms are pointed out since 50 years passed from the time Abraham drew attention to the connection between the loss complex and later depressive problems and efforts to validate the hypothesis by empirical means (Hill, 1972). In an earlier publication (Malmquist, 1975) I explained in detail what Abraham's concept of "primal parathymia" entailed for later thinking on the subject of childhood depressions. His points are summarized here to indicate how seminal his thinking was and the impact it had on subsequent theorizing, which borrowed and expanded from him.

Five independent variables were all seen as necessary for a depressive line of development to occur:

1. A constitutional element involves the area of a *predisposition* toward oral erotism. This leaves a diathesis toward excessive needs for contact, touching, etc. Early frustration and poor toleration of it result.

2. Consequently, affectionate relationships become tinged with excessive needs for affection or a correlative feeling of hurt—that the child is not getting what he or she needs. A possible offshoot is the emergence of masochistic character trends.

3. Traumatic episodes involving infantile narcissism are seen as leaving psychological scars. Such things as birth of a sibling or premature weaning were originally postulated as the types of traumas, but this laid the groundwork for much more sophisticated inquiries into the role of narcissism in depression. We now think in terms of the seemingly constant effort to repair or keep intact grandiose images (Kohut, 1971).

4. It was also postulated that the first major blow to narcissism, as an antecedent to depressive development, had to occur before the resolution of the oedipal conflict. The significance of this was that the type of triadic relationship implied by the oedipal was not yet effected, and a mixture of love and hate focused on part objects leaves a residual of ambivalence toward any person later functioning in a maternal role.

5. When subsequent blows to narcissism occur in the form of disappointments, the old mixture of hate is resurrected. The difficulty ensues from the inability to abandon ambivalent objects that have remained internalized. Later, the "stickiness" of object relationships in the depressive was seen as an extension of this context.

Subsequent work focused on intrapsychic components for some time. The expansion of theory by way of the structural model allowed the role of the superego to be introduced. When children put themselves in place of one another, they can eliminate others as well as recreate them. Wish-fulfilling creations and destructions in response to loves and hates are enacted. One part of the personality is crucial for bestowing esteem—in the form of the superego giving to the ego. Self-esteem in the depressive becomes delicately balanced because self-esteem is so dependent on approval from others. Depressive responses in the latency-age period are often triggered by minor disappointments and are associated with the primitive rage of an infant from hunger, such as the failure to satiate from sucking. This is what Rado (1928) called the failure to have a good "alimentary orgasm."

The paradigm of self-esteem based on the equivalent of "feeding" experiences leads to a heightened dependency on others. Parallel are expiatory efforts of the ego toward the superego. Since part of the hostility and rage is directed against internalized representations, when ego development is sufficient, guilt becomes a prominent part of the picture. Reparative efforts are needed to atone. "Splitting of the incorporated object" directs anger against the object or back from it. Depressive character maneuvers are observed in children of elementary school years. Interpersonal ingratiation and cautiousness with respect to expression of aggression are prominent. These are efforts of the ego toward the superego as the controller of self-esteem to reinstate a loving and beloved superego in place of one that is predominantly harsh and primitive (Schafer, 1960). The perpetuation of pressing childhood demands for approval and affection may be associated during the oedipal period with conflicts that lead to anxieties, aggression, and suffering (Gero, 1936). These thwart the pursuit of object relations without prominent ambivalence.

From psychotherapy with adult depressives, an interest in how the depressive character structure emerged was developed. Power needs were seen as part of this structure. "The discouraged child who finds that he can tyrannize best by tears will be a cry-baby, and a direct line of development leads from the cry-baby to the adult depressed patient" (Adler, 1967). Early infantile passive-aggressive activities such as pouty, whiny behavior or feeding disturbances are early manipulative techniques. The childhood prototype of the potential masochist is saying in essence, "It is giving my loved ones what they deserve if I harm myself." By adolescence this theme can be replayed endlessly by all manner of self-defeating behaviors such as use of drugs or alcohol, learning problems, and some types of delinquent activities. Similarly, the childhood prototype of the manic-depressive is one who begins everything with great enthusiasm but then gives up quickly with crying and protest behavior if brilliant success is not forthcoming. Such a child alternates between pessimistic ruminations in the realm of not having performed well and having few friends, and a feeling of self-righteous superiority.

To keep self-esteem inflated, acute sensitivity to competition arises. Demands on these children personally are resented since they feel they are being used unfairly for others' selfish interests. Consequently, such children are unwilling to give gratifications to others unless they feel they can receive themselves. If others do not give to them, they seek to extract some kind of vengeance. To them this seems like gaining justice.

Although Jacobson (1971) has written about individuals who need to betray as part of paranoid developments, I hypothesize that depressive trends are equally conspicuous. This appears connected with their seeking idealized persons or groups, from whom and through whom they hope to maintain their self-esteem. When they are disappointed, the need to hurt gains momentum. During adolescence this type of sensitivity can lead to antisocial tendencies. If these tendencies are acted on, they stem from a feeling that the acts are justified from past grievances. These traits are laid to childhood socialization experiences in which a child's needs for sincere, solicitous care were unfulfilled. Manipulative efforts toward peers and authorities are repeated patterns for dealing with extractive and manipulative parental figures. "He has been deprived, and he feels gyped and is angrily determined to get what is rightfully his. . . . In this defiant, stubborn, angry, begrudging battle of something-for-nothing, he loses the enjoyments of adolescence, of young adulthood, and of later adulthood" (Bonime, 1966). How valid are these observations of the childhood depressive as manipulator? These character traits are observed in children, and they acquire increasing sophistication with use. However, theorizing that makes manipulative aspects of personality development the crux of the depressive personality underemphasizes other key elements. The "depressive character" is not synonymous with the "neurotic character."

OBJECT RELATIONS AND DEPRESSIONS

Theories about the development and maintenance of "object relations, attachment, bonding, and dependency needs" have implications for the depression-prone child. Confirmation or disproof of theories takes place through observations in the naturalistic setting where children develop since that is where depressive affect originates. Confusion has emerged from different usages for all these terms (Ainsworth, 1969). Workers from different disciplines employing different psychological frameworks have accentuated the problem. Some have worked in nurseries, others in nursery schools, and yet others have carried out experimental work. None of these sources derive their theories from clinical work, which provides still another source for ideas about object relations.

"Object relations" is the term most clinicians use in referring to the agents who gratify or deprive an infant. In this context, the infant is seen as dependent. "Instinct theory" conceptualizes the object against whom drives are carried out. Discriminatory and perceptual capacities are diffuse in the young infant with little cognitive appreciation. Rather, an awareness of tensions is experienced psychologically as narcissistic disequilibrium. As more ego functions develop, an increasing capacity to distinguish his "self" and body from others permits distinctions between objects and their types of responses. This is not seen simply as a passive registry but rather as an active organization or seeking of stimulation (Gewirtz, 1973).

"Object constancy" permits images, qualities, and affects associated with objects to be maintained in their absence. It is not confined to states of satisfaction or deprivation. Through this internalization, the preobject child establishes the permanence of objects. However, this ongoing presence of introjects as a continuing psychological representation has two sides. These introjects can be supportive and bestow self-esteem, or they can be critical or punitive.

These formulations have analogues with social learning theory aspects that focus on "dependency" as a secondary (acquired) drive. Primary satisfaction was used, along with which incidentally went the developing awareness of an "object." When an infant's physiological needs were satisfied, he learned who it was who gratified him. Social needs were acquired as by-products. This drive-reduction theory of dependency has been criticized. If behavior attributable to "drives" can be accounted for in terms of "reinforcing stimuli" operating in the environment, behavior is contingent on environmental reinforcement. The environment rather than the organism becomes primary. These stimuli are events occurring subsequent to behaviors that are operantly emitted and controlled by instrumental conditioning. "Dependency" is viewed neither as a reflection of a drive nor as a trait, but simply as certain learned behaviors. The "object" is significant only as a particular stimulus object. Dependency is linked to objects, but it is not restricted to the context of someone who is providing food or reducing tension. Rather than an emphasis on the "rewards" provided by objects in the service of drive reduction, stress is on the salience of objects. Salience attaches to an object's "attention-getting" characteristics or through an increased frequency of exposure. As an example, sheep become attached to television sets when isolated from other animals but in constant propinquity to an operating set (Cairns, 1966*b*). An implication for a theory of depressions is present here. Separation from a salient object should have no more significance than setting in motion a process of relearning to whatever new object is currently salient (Cairns, 1966*a*). Over time, strength of attachment should thus directly wane, but in practice we do not find this so. It is mentioned to illustrate how some experimental findings can be incongruent with clinical work and also with the experience of continuity in psychological life. It does demonstrate a type of theorizing divorced from a framework where account can be taken of internalized neurophysiological structures as well as cognitive and affective processes.

In addition to a secondary drive theory or environmental operants, a third alternative for the development of object relations has its roots in biology and ethology. Developing an attachment in itself is seen as *primary*. The infant is seen with a built-in need for an object in its own right apart from drive reduction. Attachment develops apart from feeding experiences but also where "releasing" stimuli of many types activate the process. Internal neurophysiological and neurohumoral states are the "primers" operating on a genetic substate that has the potential to activate attachments. Learning operates to reinforce or lessen certain attachment behaviors. The "attachment process" originating in the organism is distinguished from the various "attachment behaviors" mediating it. Although the latter are overt and hence more easily measurable, they are not the same as the basis for these behaviors. The deceptiveness of relying on external behaviors is seen in assessing a child who clings and weeps as necessarily more depressed than a child who sits forlornly with little animation. Conversely, more demonstrative attachment behaviors do not imply greater attachment. Hidden in these formulations regarding object ties is the possible need to rethink our hypotheses regarding "oral mechanisms" and depressions. The emphasis in attachment theory is that the system underlying attachment, with its crucial significance for social relations, is not a consequence of the original feeding prototype. It is its own discrete and endogenous system.

BOWLBY AND KLEIN

Bowlby's (1958) ideas about "instinctual response systems" in humans as contributing to attachment should be noted. These ideas maintain the proximity of children to maternal objects. Attachment occurs by way of certain behavioral systems being activated for five response patterns: sucking, clinging, following, crying, and smiling. Evolutionary processes elicit these responses, and they interact with principal figures in the environment (Bowlby, 1969). Many arguments persist regarding the functions served by attachment behaviors. A prominent criticism is that no postulates about drives are needed and reliance on control systems suffices. Another criticism is that studying attachment behaviors in terms of manifest behaviors is not actually studying the internal psychological processes involved in attachment and object relations (Engel, 1971).

Many clinicians rely on object relations theory for their theory of childhood depressions. Melanie Klein (1948) postulated introjective-projective processes occurring from birth onward. This is criticized as telescoping into the first year certain psychological processes that are ordinarily spread throughout childhood. The "depressive position" is connected with the loss accompanying weaning between 3 and 12 months. This is seen as a normal and unavoidable developmental situation, derived from an earlier "paranoid position." Superego structuralization during the first year is believed related to feelings of possessiveness and destructiveness toward a parental object rather than incestuous wishes emerging several years later.

The depressive position develops in moving from a "part" to a "whole" object relationship. In the predepressive position only relations to parts of objects, such as a breast, are believed present. During the depressive position the mother is perceived as a whole object. This permits ambivalence and accompanying anxiety about the loss of the entire love object. The infant experiences a guilty anxiety with a need to preserve this good object which calls forth magical devices. Reparative work is in the service of making amends to undo sadistic attacks on introjective objects; parallel to these intrapsychic maneuvers are actual situations where the excited infant achieves instinctual gratification, such as during feeding. Since the object "attacked" is the same one providing security, there is the potential for despair. The infantile depressive position is related to this potential since later depressions occur over loss of objects with fear of abandonment and loss. The contrast is the security where internalized objects are accepted as bestowing love and security. An individual can accumulate memories of experiences felt to be good so that they become part of himself and are assimilated into the ego. In this way the actual mother gradually becomes less necessary (Winnicott, 1954).

GRIEF AND MOURNING

Grief and mourning in infancy have been discussed by Bowlby (1960*a,b;* 1961*a,b;* 1973) in connection with activation of attachment behaviors when maternal figures continue to be unavailable. This work is important regarding the nature of childhood bereavement. It also generates hypotheses regarding the pathogenic potential of mourning processes when reactions to losses take a pathological turn. Removal of young children from their mothers initiates successive psychological phases: numbness, protest, despair, and detachment. Each phase has an accompanying parallel response of separation anxiety, grief and mourning, and defense, although they all operate as part of a unitary process. "Mourning" refers to a psychological process set in motion by loss of a loved object, whereas "grief" is the parallel subjective state in such a loss. "Depression" is the affective state when mourning is occurring, as distinguished from the clinical syndrome of melancholia. One of Bowlby's postulates is that loss of a mother figure between 6 months and 3 to 4 years of age has a high degree of pathogenic potential for subsequent personality development because of the occurrence of mourning processes.

Protesting behavior is manifested in crying, motoric restlessness, and angry efforts to regain the lost object by demands for its return. This sows the seeds for later psychopathology. Subsequent disorganization with painful despair hopefully leads to a reorganization in connection with relinquishing the image of the lost object with the help of new objects. Anger is believed essential for efforts to recover the lost object. Yearning is mixed with repeated disappointments in not recovering the object that is lost. Grief is connected with an irretrievable loss, whereas separation anxiety is a response to a situation in which hope persists that the loss is not irretrievable.

Persistence of efforts to regain experienced losses can have four possible types of pathological outcomes: (1) Unconscious yearnings to recover lost objects persist. These seem surprising to clinicians since there is an absence of grief. (2) Angry reproaches are hurled against the self and other objects to attain a reunion. Displacement of reproaches occurs in which inappropriate objects are used or mourned at a distance. Development to the level at which anger can be directed against the self as a psychological process is an index that guilt is experienced. Guilt is generated through reality-based realizations that the child has played a role in the loss or through fantasies that the object was destroyed. Psychopathological displacement is owing to prolongation of anger without direct expression. Chronicity itself leads to a waning of affectionate components. (3) Absorption in caring for others who are suffering is substituted for grieving oneself by way of projective identification and vicarious mourning. This should be suspected when a child is plagued by "bad luck" or indulges in compulsive pitying of others. (4) Denial of the permanency of object loss operating on a conscious level necessitates a "split in the ego." Acute losses have a greater tendency to result in such denial. Children are particularly prone to react to losses in this manner. Losses predispose the child to character changes that leave him in a state of readiness to evoke similar reactions when subsequent developmental, psychological, or environmental losses occur. This process is analogous to being exposed to an allergen.

Bowlby's theories are not automatically accepted. He once held that no qualitative difference existed between mourning in children and that in adults on the basis that their behavior appeared similar. However, Bowlby's position was later clarified in holding that pathological mourning persists in children because of their failure to engage in normal mourning processes when the object is lost (Bowlby, 1963). A review of the literature concludes that children, in contrast to adults, do not go through a stage of mourning in which they gradually experience a painful detachment from the inner representation of the person who has died (Miller, 1971). Rather, a complex set of defensive phenomena functions to deny what has occurred, and this has a pathogenic potential.

There is a need to consider differences in successive developmental stages and how they affect psychological reactions to object loss (Freud, 1960). When young children grieve, they experience a "hurt" rather than undergo the same psychological processes as adults. Some describe this in terms of a lack of developmental readiness to mourn before adolescence.

Until he has undergone what we may call the trial mourning of adolescence, he is unable to mourn. Once he has lived through the painful, protracted decathecting of the first love objects, he can repeat the process when circumstances of external loss require a similar renunciation. When such loss occurs, we may picture the individual who has been initiated into mourning through adolescence confronting himself with the preconscious question: 'Can I bear to give up someone I love so much?' The answer follows: 'Yes, I can bear it—I have been through it once before.' Before the trial mourning of adolescence has been undergone, a child making the same tentative beginning of reality testing in regard to a major object loss is threatened with the prospect of overwhelming panic and retreats into defensive denial in the way we have observed (Wolfenstein, 1966).

EXTENSIONS OF OBJECT LOSS INTO DEPRESSIVE PRONENESS

Object loss as a concept has been expanded far beyond that of a literal loss to include distortions in object relationships. Depressive consequences can be subtle and not show up in the form of gross disturbance but lie in wait until some unspecified future time. Depressed moods in mothers during the first 2 years after birth create a tendency to similar moods in the children which later become manifest (Freud, 1965). Fusion with a depressed mother induces the mood disturbance in children, especially in children who live an "as if" existence in which they perceive themselves as necessary for validation of parental needs. The liability is the threat of abandonment if they are not validating (Brodey, 1965). Serious and chronic preoccupations in the parents leave little room for spontaneous curiosity and interaction with the children in their world. Pessimistic moods in the parents induce feelings of failure in children whereby children feel they are somehow responsible for the predicament of the parents. Depressed and worried parents interfere with the freedom of children to play and test their environment free from apprehension about their parents. Similarly, parents staving off their depressed moods by extreme and unpredictable activity and periodic overstimulating play with a child contribute to the depressive outlook of the child (Davidson, 1968).

Clinical work reveals that not all children with "narcissistic vulnerabilities" have lost an external object. Relevant are the developmental lines striving to attain object constancy in efforts to achieve separation and individuation. Individuation gives rise to a period of increased psychomotor activity from 10 to 18 months in which the mood is believed to be one of infantile elation. Actively leaving and returning with a maternal readiness for the infant doing this are steps toward acquiring an internal object constancy. "Giving up" the fusion promotes individuation and is a step toward lowering magical maneuverings (Mahler, 1961). Depressive moods are generated by a child's relinquishment of a belief in his omnipotence and a feeling that the parents are withholding power from him. These moods manifest themselves by separation and grief reactions marked by temper tantrums, continual attempts to woo or coerce the mother, and then periods of giving up in despair for a while. In some cases there is impotent resignation and surrender that may have a marked masochistic coloring. On the other hand, discontentment and anger can persist after a short period of grief and sadness (Mahler, 1966). The natural history of these early mood states in the preschool child reveals many of them giving way to premature earnestness ("little adults"). An undue seriousness indicates precocious superego formation. Other signs of failing to attain object constancy with respect to mood are marked ambivalence, precocious overidentification, pseudo-self-sufficiency, and a flattened overt emotional spontaneity.

The evolution of a depreciated self-concept is a major predisposing influence in the formation of a depressive nucleus in a child. Emotional distantness on the part of family members puts children into a nuclear conflict. They are not in a position to understand or appraise the reasons for this treatment of them. Nor do parents comprehend the innumerable ways their reactions to children are manifested. Early self-derogatory cognitions emerge in the form of negative self-cognitions, to wit, "I am no good." These are not confined to major areas of failings but are carried out with respect to many minor failings initially. Self-evaluations as intrinsically defective or disappointments as a person emerge. Feelings of loneliness and abandonment proceed to states of despair and general incompetence. An adolescent born with a congenital harelip that precipitated a hospitalized depression in her mother reported being distant from her mother during her childhood years. She had heard her mother tell her aunts that she would never take a chance on another pregnancy (which she didn't). Losing herself in books worked up to a point as did compulsive study habits. They were not sufficient to contain her depression after her mother's death when her regrets centered on verbalizations that she would now never know her mother and her anger about this.

Because of how seriously these young children view life, anything less than perfection in them raises the possibility of abandonment (Reich, 1960). The internal threat is far more severe than that from the parents. Although parental anger has limits, that of the superego may not. Unattainable ideals are related to this perfectionism. This manifests itself in a vulnerability to seek out hero figures who possess the perfect characteristics lacking in the potentially depressed child. In children this is seen in overevaluating others as more competent, more popular, brighter, etc. However, heroes are always subject to cause disillusion: then instead of being idealized, the heroes are criticized and all their faults are overemphasized (Main, 1971). One of the benefits of an accepting therapist for these children is that in the therapeutic setting the children do not have to earn acceptance. In time, however, the idealizing transference with the therapist needs handling.

Within our expanding knowledge of the developmental role of narcissism in children lies another key to understanding the impact of loss on children. Repeated rebuffs or losses are reacted to as confirmations that a significant person did not value them and that they are therefore unworthy (Rochlin, 1965). How they feel becomes increasingly sensitized to transient environmental approvals from other children, which leaves them narcissistically vulnerable. Pushed to an extreme this can lead to deficits in reality testing. This is in accord with the principle that narcissism increases as the importance of real objects diminishes. Yet such withdrawal is unsatisfactory to children and leads to "restitutive" attempts to restore real relationships.

In young children, losses are partially met by an increase in narcissism, and also by their capacity for adaptation by acceptance of substitute objects. Loss of self-esteem as a response to loss is not thought to appear until a structural division of mental activity has been accomplished. By then object constancy has been attained so mourning as a process of detachment from inner representations can occur. Only when an object has attained value does its loss lead to self-devaluation. Aggression directed against the self is witnessed in masochistic phenomena as part of a depressive picture. When an object becomes important the child becomes concerned with the question, "Who will love me when I am left?" and the answer, "No one may want you" (Rochlin, 1961). A child who feels depleted and devalued as an object does not conceptualize himself as worth much.

Mood variations are another accompaniment. Somatic manifestations are the template for similar symptoms as the children grow up, and these symptoms appear as hypochondriasis, motor restlessness, sleep upsets, and gastrointestinal complaints. Children's moods have three main characteristics (Jacobson, 1957): (1) affective manifestations are more intense than in adults because of insufficient ego-superego controls; (2) mood swings are briefer— they change rapidly because of the instability of object relations and the greater readiness of children to accept substitute objects and gratifications; (3) the affective range in children is more limited than that of adults because of lack of ego differentiation. When a propensity toward pathological mood disturbance develops, there is actually less variety and spontaneity of moods. A more exaggerated quality is presently seen in persistent forlornness and sadness or exaggerated excitement.

LATENCY-AGE DEPRESSIONS

An increasing amount has been written about depressive responses in young children and animals on one level, and about the more flamboyant behavior of depressed adolescents on the other. Yet, children from 5 years of age to puberty may actually comprise the most hidden group in terms of incidence. Investigators are confused about how thwarted dependency needs, physical illnesses, and losses induce depressive reactions in this age group (Rie, 1966). Although internalized conflict creates possibilities for many types of neurotic conflicts, not all feel that the concepts elaborated about depression are applicable to children (Koran, 1975). Confusion is compounded by the "latent" manifestations of depression at this age in which there is often an absence of the overt symptoms associated with depressions. Hence, crying, verbalized self-condemnations, and overt expressions of guilt are not the primary symptom picture. Parental use of denial regarding one of their children who appears sad or unhappy further masks true incidence.

We know from clinical and developmental work that latency is no more quiescent than any other period of life. What adds complexity is the emergence of a control system that can be quite variable. Superego functioning is particularly prone to become involved in conflict. It is common to observe children placing severe demands on themselves. For some this is owing to immaturity in their control systems; for others it is a projection of aggression onto internalized representations.

An increasing number of articles have appeared referring to depressed children. The symptom pictures described vary widely and are based on differing criteria for inclusion as part of a depressive syndrome. Given our early stage in delineating a picture for the various faces of childhood depression, it would seem premature to try to set rigid limits on what should be included and excluded in this diagnosis. We could achieve only a false reassurance that a high degree of reliability exists. It is not apparent that, even for the most traditional of organic medical illnesses and diagnostic procedures, a high degree of reliability exists (Koran, 1975). However, to increase our sophistication and carry out research, we need some system to progress now that the consensus seems to be that children do indeed become depressed. A working classification for the diverse manifestations of childhood depression is possible. Although age is part of the picture, other contributory factors are also listed: (1) deprivation-type syndromes (anaclitic depressions); (2) physical illnesses (primary, such as in diabetes, or reactive, e.g., a response to disease); (3) separation-individuation problems; (4) object losses; (5) overdeveloped ego-ideal systems; (6) depressive equivalents; and (7) cyclothymic mood disturbances.

How does the depressed child appear? As with depressions in different age groups, a myriad of pictures is possible. Although there is a confluence in some children, the signs and symptoms vary widely. Some of these observations are made from children in intensive therapy, whereas others are from children on inpatient units and yet others are from those in outpatient departments or court settings. Some of the observations are from a retrospective awareness of a symptom picture in midchildhood by adolescents or adults who realize during therapy how depressed they were at that time (Sandler and Joffe, 1965). Drawn from these sources, the following is a composite picture of how a depressed child would appear based on our present state of knowledge (Malmquist, 1971a,b).

1. A general picture of a sad, depressed, or unhappy looking child may be present. The child does not complain of unhappiness, or even exhibit awareness of it, but rather conveys a psychomotor behavioral picture of sadness.
2. Withdrawal and inhibition with little interest in any activity may be most prominent. Listlessness gives an impression of boredom or physical illness and often leads an observer to conclude that the child must have some concealed physical illness.
3. Somatizing takes the form of physical pain (headaches, abdominal complaints, dizziness), insomnia, sleeping or eating disturbances—"depressive equivalents."
4. A quality of discontent is prominent. An initial impression is that the child is dissatisfied and experiences little pleasure, and in time the clinician gathers the added impression that others—even an examiner who has barely met the child—are somehow responsible for his plight. In some

cases blame is cast on others in the sense of easily criticizing other children.

5. A sense of feeling rejected or unloved is present. There is a readiness to turn away from disappointing objects.
6. Negative self-concepts reflect cognitive patterns of illogically concluding that they are worthless, etc. (Beck, 1972).
7. Reports are made of observations of low frustration tolerance and irritability; this is coupled with self-punitive behavior when goals are not attained.
8. Although the child conveys a sense of needing or wanting comfort, reassurance is then accepted as his due, or he remains dissatisfied and discontent although he is often ignorant as to why.
9. Reversal of affect is revealed in clowning and dealing with underlying depressive feelings by foolish or provocative behavior to detract from assets or achievements.
10. Blatant attempts to deny feelings of helplessness and hopelessness are seen in the Charlie Brown syndrome, modeled after the cartoon character of a boy from 7 to 9 years who avoids confronting his despair and disillusionment by being self-deprecatory and then springing back with hope (Symonds, 1968). These actions indicate a hope that self-deprecations, avoidance of rewards, dedicated effort, and other examples of being "good" will lead to rewards that are just—perhaps when one grows up or at least in the hereafter. Hope enables children to avoid the more overt manifestations of depressive pessimism seen in the adult when disillusionment occurs.
11. Provocative behavior stirs angry responses in others and leads others to use the child as a focus for their own disappointments. Such scapegoating indicates suffering, which leads to descriptions of the child as a "born loser." Difficulties in handling aggression may be a frequent reason for referral.
12. The children exhibit tendencies to passivity and expect others to anticipate their needs. Since this is frequently impossible, they may express their anger by passive-aggressive techniques.
13. Sensitivity and high standards with a readiness to condemn themselves for failures are common. There is a preference to be harsh and self-critical. This appears as an attempt to avoid conflict associated with hostility by in effect saying, "I don't blame you—only myself." In some this extends to the point of feeling they are so bad they should be dead (McConville, 1973).
14. Obsessive compulsive behavior is seen in connection with other types of regressive, magical activities.
15. Episodic acting-out behaviors are used as a defensive maneuver to avoid experiencing painful feelings associated with depression.

The phenomenological experience of depression-prone children presents an intriguing picture. In some ways they appear as caricatures of the adult intellectual who intensely worries about the state of mankind. With children, the worry is about their own worthwhileness. They convey an inner hesitancy that shows up as a fear of commitment—be it in peer relationships or activities. This seems to correlate with an uncertainty about others remaining reliable and steadfast. Clinicians sense a cautious seeking for attachments during therapy and in reports of their daily life. In contrast to a schizoid child who prefers his withdrawal, the depressed child hungers for a relationship but he is doubtful about its sustainingness. Although the child is externally forlorn and sad, he is usually unaware of the reasons for his altered moods or why he periodically reacts as he does.

Affective states of nostalgia and self-pity do not seem present developmentally until age 3 to 4. At that time children verbalize their feelings when someone leaves them and is missed. Sensitive observers sense mild depressive affect when a parent, pet, or friend is absent for more than a short period. Displays of narcissistic mortification may amuse adults. Thus, a 4-year-old may refuse to participate in an activity which he enjoys a great deal when something is denied him or he is reprimanded. Miscarried attempts to hurt frustrating and controlling objects by not cooperating in some activity pleasing the other party is a possible outcome. All manner of masochistic phenomena may follow, such as learning problems and putting oneself at a disadvantage with other children. A 12-year-old girl turns down a role in a school play because she is afraid her friend will not be invited. A boy of 11 holds back in a race for fear of winning. The line between altruism and masochism can be quite thin. When these behaviors are described by the child and one senses an accompanying affect of self-pity for the sacrifice, the actions are probably masochistic. The subjects of success phobias and those wrecked by success are relevant. Some children can become quite skillful in arranging situations in which they can feel offended. For example, a child who wants a certain job in school can manage by reticence and concealing to keep her assets unknown, while a child with lesser ability but more assertiveness obtains the job. The former child can then nurse her wounds in solitude but experience hurt and mortification.

A frequent pattern that cannot be ignored as an antecedent is the presence in the home of an adult who becomes depressed periodically. The emotional tone of sadness, hurt, and loneliness in the adult leaves a tone of sadness in the child. This could be based on identification with a depressed parent or on using depression as a defense to control rage that has not been handled otherwise (Poznaski and Zrull, 1970).

From this background, children with clinical depressions appear as sufferers. Some rely on somatizing processes or endless appearances at physicians' offices for problems that cannot be explained physically. In many ways these are varieties of "masked depressions" that are subsumed under the category of endogenousness for adults (Lopez, 1972). The most frequent somatic symptoms in children are headaches, dizziness, cephalalgias, nausea, abdominal pain, or wandering pains in different parts of the body. In two successive series of 100 children investigated for recurrent abdominal pain ("little bellyachers"), only 8% and 6%, respectively, were found to have an organically explainable defect (Apley, 1959). Not only abdominal complaints, but also anorexia, pruritus, and migraine headaches have been viewed as depressive equivalents in children (Sperling, 1959). Severe encopresis has been considered a depressive equivalent in children when there is open expression of aggression. Similarly, enuresis has been viewed as part of a symptom complex in a depressed child in whom genitourinary evaluations and cystoscopy reveal no organic pathology (Frommer, 1968).

Depressed children can be "loners," not in the sense of schizoidia, but rather because their worries and preoccupations interfere with their engaging with others as they are capable of. Feeling lonely may result in teasing and sadistic behavior. Vicarious pleasure in seeing others commit errors or injure themselves then becomes part of the mechanism for diverting self-critical attack on themselves. Abrupt shifts in behavior in a child should raise a question of depression. Thus, a previously alert child who shows signs of withdrawal, apathy, or inability to study and lack of interest most often makes people think of a physical source, but these symptoms are equally compatible with depression. A previously outgoing and carefree child who grows quiet and preoccupied, or a conforming child with obsessional tendencies who shows more mood variations or episodes of "delinquent" behavior also qualifies. A superior student whose achievement reflects high aspirations and ideals is likely to react with depressive manifestations when rewards for his hard work are not forthcoming or when maintenance of earlier overachievements becomes difficult. Vulnerability in such children lies in their overachievement and overconscientiousness. Obsessional activities in the depressed child represent efforts to compensate for feelings of helplessness. Jarvis (1965) noted an association between loneliness and compulsivity in children in which the compulsions served as a defense against sadness and loss. These feelings are evoked in response to a pattern of "withdrawn mothering," in which physical needs are met but the absence of the mother makes her unable to gratify some basic psychological needs of the child.

Hyperactive and restless behavior in the depressed child seem paradoxical. It is interesting that these were the symptoms of depression noted in a 1931 report by Kasanin. Hyperkinesis is seen in a variety of disturbances, varying from cerebral dysfunction to defensive maneuvers. Hyperkinetic behavior in the depressed child may be similar psychodynamically to hypomanic activity in adults who are warding off depressive feelings. Hyperactive behavior, like antisocial behavior, brings parental condemnation and allows the parent to focus on such behavior while long-standing hostilities are ignored. An increasing amount of clinical work confirms a viewpoint that certain forms of antisocial behavior or acting out in children are a response to a depressive core. In his original monograph, Bowlby (1951) felt there was a specific connection between prolonged early deprivation and the development of a personality with shallow relationships with other people, poor impulse control, and the development of an "affectionless, psychopathic character." There is continued need for clinical documentation of the relationship between depressions and persistent criminality, which is so often bypassed in group statistics on crime (Cormier, 1966).

DEPRESSED CHILDREN AND ACTING OUT

Although it may be unnecessary, there will be an opening caveat. No claim is made that all deficits in object relations give rise to a depressive nucleus which then leads to antisocial behavior. Indeed, if unmitigated hate exists toward an object and its introject, more primitive emotions of hate and rage not tempered by ambivalence occur (Berman, 1959). Nor does guilt predominate in this latter type of situation. This type of antisocial development associated with impulsive behavior is not going to be discussed further, and it is mentioned simply before we proceed to how neurotically depressed children resort to acting-out behavior.

Depressed children experience losses as a painful discomfort that makes up part of their depressive core. Their acting out is related either to anxiety about object loss (separation) or to sadness that can progress to despair if they feel the object or part-object will not be recovered. In some of these children, anger related to this predicament can take the form of attacks against people or the environment because of loss of a dependent object or frustration about hunger for an object. Neurotically depressed children behave as though they have already performed in an unacceptable manner, as though either some unacceptable impulse has been carried out or they have somehow failed (Brenner, 1975). The importance of narcissism has been mentioned.

A depressed child with this burden of guilt may also act out in order to secure punishment. This is the model Franz Alexander (1930) elaborated as a concomitant of the neurotic character. Such children tend to be whiny or nagging, or if more deeply guilty they can carry out acts of vandalism or arson and then feel relieved.

An example is that of a previously well-behaved but progressively sad 10-year-old girl. As an only child, she had many mixed unresolved oedipal romance feelings toward her father and guilt feelings toward her mother; she found herself becoming quieter and sadder as latency wore on. In retrospect, her parents agreed with this but said that it had occurred so insidiously that they had done no more than comment on it once to each other. One night, their next door neighbor's home, occupied by a childless newly married couple, was broken into through an open window. This 10-year-old scratched profane words over the walls with lipstick, and then slashed the bedding and mattress with a knife. Although the neighborhood and police at first thought a local sex maniac had been on the loose, to her horror the mother discovered the used lipstick tube in the child's bedroom. The child subsequently felt bad, but she also felt less sad than over the previous months.

Resistance to a treatment approach that sets limits to acting out is needed since this requires the child to experience the underlying depression with the therapist. What first appears then is often somatic complaints. Self-destructive behavior often parallels strong guilt and self-hate. Aggressive behavior is used to avoid depressed feelings, especially when there is a direct threat to the integrity of the child. Situations in which children cannot deny their cravings for affection or those in which past feelings of worthlessness become overwhelming pose such threats (Burks and Harrison, 1962). It is not just that acting out and delinquent patterns represent attempts at coping with some type of depressive nucleus. Further questions arise about the nature of distortions in development that have occured when the ego permits the aggression to be acted out during a childhood depression (Kaufman, 1955; Kaufman et al., 1963). To what extent are some of these components of the depressive character structure reversible? How modifiable will they be by therapy, or should we view them as fixed traits that will characterize an individual throughout life?

Acting-out behavior has particular psychodynamic and social meanings. Some believe that acting out is a primary defense in a majority of depressive individuals. As noted, this does not exclude its presence with different diagnostic categories, such as impulse-ridden characters, those with defective socialization patterns, antisocial personalities, or as part of a schizophrenic process. In part, the problem is a conceptual one since "primary theorists" view depressive affect as crucial to whatever overt diagnostic features are present. By latency, a progressive pattern of hatred and destructive behavior in fantasy, play, and overt behavior is possible. The narcissistic basis and ambivalence in object ties is striking. However, therapeutic work that deals with the personality structure beneath the external aggressive display sees a denigrated self-concept. The child and parent are both mutually identifying with the "bad" parts of each other. This reinforces feelings of worthlessness. Repetitive play themes or fantasies relating to destroying bad things are followed by magically reconstituting them. For some depressed children, the fantasies are acted out and the fascinating question is why this occurs in some of these children.

The formulations of Therese Benedek (1956) regarding the "depressive constellation" are relevant here. When oral demands and frustrations of children reactivate similar conflicts in the mother, the transactions between them give rise to an "ambivalent core." Child and mother interact on a projective and introjective bipolar basis of aggression in an attempt to escape from feelings of being a "bad child" and "bad mother." The model is that of identification of the mother "backward" with her own child, who is reenacting the provocative role of the mother as child. The hypothesis is that certain parents have had childhood experiences that heighten this ambivalent core. A pattern of reinforcing hostility is mutually set in motion and gains momentum. The child feels estranged and angry, and these feelings are superimposed on the disappointment of the parent. In turn, the parent feels justified in condemning the angry, sullen child, who develops feelings of shame that lead to increasing distance. Repetitive acting out then ensues with the original and now concealed depressive nucleus being the impelling motive to these patterns.

This affect of shame is so powerful and painful for a child to deal with that the ego erects a set of defenses to handle it. How does this affect arise in connection with a depressed child? Secondly, what is the relationship of shame to acting out? Part of the depressive complex is a failure to live up to inflated ego ideals with a resultant vulnerability to believe more readily that one has failed. In such a failure complex, shame is one of the leading affects. The child experiences this failure in interpersonal terms of being criticized, ridiculed, and excluded by others, and in ego terms as one of feeling the pain of humiliation.

But then why do some children not simply rest here and accept their humiliated selves? Some do just that, and they become part of the group of chronic losers. The result is that they accept a picture of inadequacy as their norm. This solution appears related to the threat of greater pain if they do not so acquiesce in that image. On some level this maintains the facsimile of a relationship against the threat of total dissolution.

However, this type of acquiescence may be too painful for some children caught in such a conflict. Blame for their disappointing performances may be projected onto others. This projection can be quite forceful if the parental figures join in with the child. In fact, it may lead to a rare experience of togetherness on an emotional level for the child. Hence, a depreciated and depressed child who blames poor teaching for his failures to get the As his parents want may be joined by his parents in the attack. This is often quite effective since school personnel often take the role of the culprit by accommodating this type of criticism.

If these measures of alleviating the painful ego state of shame do not work for the child, he may resort to more open aggressive attacks. A child shamed for his deficient academic performance may act out his impulses in a classroom or more brazenly by writing profanity on the bathroom walls, for example. A child criticized by his gym teacher, as well as by his parents, for a poor performance in a competitive event may begin to leave feces scattered around the school. An 11-year-old girl subject to disdain by her parents for not gaining acceptance by the right social group in her school may organize her own clique. As its leader, she may manage in turn to reject many other girls who want to be accepted by her group. These temporary triumphs do little to assuage her nagging sense of shame and inadequacy. Although previously seen as a child wanting acceptance quite badly but uncertain about herself, she is now seen as an angry, embittered, and cunning child. Just as there are "criminals from a sense of guilt" (Levin, 1971), "criminals from a sense of shame" have been pointed out. By adolescence more borderline delinquency if not criminal acts are probable from this depressive framework.

SUMMARY

This chapter has surveyed some of the salient problems in depressive phenomena beginning in infancy and proceeding into latency. The multifarious clinical manifestations that occur from infancy up to adolescence are often ignored. They have been dealt with from a critical perspective involving theoretical problems present in evolving a coherent clinical picture. A systematic set of signs and symptoms is necessary if any assessment of depressed children is to be meaningful. Developmental aspects of moods, reactive mood swings, and clinical symptom pictures have been differentiated. By the time that a relatively fixed style of responses to losses or to disappointments environmentally, or with respect to the child's own ego ideal, has been developed, the predispostion for clinical depressions has been established. The depressive cycle has then been initiated, and it is a difficult process to dislodge.

REFERENCES

Abraham, K. (1911) Notes on the psycho-analytical investigation and treatment of manic-depressive insanity and allied conditions. In: *On Character and Libido Development*. New York, W. W. Norton, pp. 15–34, 1966.

Abraham, K. A short study of the development of the libido, viewed in the light of mental disorders (1924). In: *On Character and Libido Development*. New York, W. W. Norton, pp. 67–150, 1966.

Adler, K. A. Adler's individual psychology. In B. B. Wolman (ed.): *Psychoanalytic Techniques*. New York, Basic Books, pp. 299–337, 1967.

Ainsworth, M. D. S. Object relations, dependency and attachment: A theoretical review of the infant-mother relationship. *Child Dev.*, 40:969–1025, 1969.

Alexander, F. The neurotic character (1930). In: *The Scope of Psychoanalysis*. New York, Basic Books, pp. 56–89, 1961.

Apley, J. *The Child with Abdominal Pain*. Springfield, Ill., Charles C. Thomas, 1959.

Baldesserini, R. Frequency of diagnosis of schizophrenia and affective disorder from 1944–1968. *Am. J. Psychiatry*, 127:759–763, 1970.

Beck, A. T. *Depression Causes and Treatment*. Philadelphia, University of Pennsylvania Press, 1972.

Benedek, T. Towards the biology of the depressive constellation. *J. Am. Psychoanal. Assoc.*, 4:389–427, 1956.

Berger, M., and Passingham, R. E. Early experience and other environmental factors: An overview. In H. J. Eysenck (ed.): *Handbook of Abnormal Psychology, Ed. 2*. London, Pittman, 1973.

Berman, S. Antisocial character disorder: Its etiology and relationship to delinquency. *Am. J. Orthopsychiatry*, 29:612–621, 1959.

Bonime, W. The psychodynamics of neurotic depression. In S. Arieti (ed.): *American Handbook of Psychiatry, Vol. 3*. New York, Basic Books, pp. 239–255, 1966.

Bowlby, J. *Maternal Care and Mental Health, Ed. 2*. Geneva, World Health Organization, 1951.

Bowlby, J. The nature of the child's tie to the mother. *Int. J. Psychoanal.*, 39:350–373, 1958.

Bowlby, J. Grief and mourning in infancy and early childhood. *Psychoanal. Study Child*, 15:9–52, 1960a.

Bowlby, J. Separation anxiety. *Int. J. Psychoanal.*, 41:89–113, 1960b.

Bowlby, J. Childhood mourning and its implication for psychiatry. *Am. J. Psychiatry*, 118:481–498, 1961a.

Bowlby, J. Processes of mourning. *Int. J. Psychoanal.*, 42:317–340, 1961*b*.

Bowlby, J. Pathological mourning and childhood mourning. *J. Am. Psychoanal. Assoc.*, 11:500–541, 1963.

Bowlby, J. *Attachment and Loss, Vol. 1.* New York, Basic Books, 1969.

Bowlby, J. *Attachment and Loss, Vol. 2.* New York, Basic Books, 1973.

Brenner, C. Affects and psychic conflict. *Psychoanal. Q.* 44:5–28, 1975.

Brodey, W. M. On the dynamics of narcissism. I. Externalization and early ego development. *Psychoanal. Study Child,* 20:165–193, 1965.

Burks, H. L., and Harrison S. I. Aggressive behavior as a means of avoiding depression. *Am. J. Orthopsychiatry,* 32:416–422, 1962.

Burlingham, D., and Freud, A. *Infants Without Families.* London, Allen & Unwin, 1943.

Cairns, R. B. Attachment behavior of mammals. *Psychol. Rev.,* 23:409–426, 1966*a*.

Cairns, R. B. Development, maintenance, and extinction of social attachment behavior in sheep. *J. Comp. Physiol. Psychol.,* 62:298–306, 1966*b*.

Coddington, R. D. Study of an infant with gastric fistula and her normal twin. *Psychosom. Med.,* 30:172–192, 1968.

Cormier, B. M. Depression and persistent criminality. *Can. Psychiatry Assoc. J. Suppl.,* 11:208–220, 1966.

Davidson, J. Infantile depression in a "normal" child. *J. Am. Acad. Child Psychiatry,* 7:522–535, 1968.

Diagnostic and Statistical Manual of Mental Disorders, Ed. 2. Washington, D.C., American Psychiatric Association, 1968.

Eisenberg, L. Problems for the biopsychology of development. In E. Tobach, L. R. Aronson, and E. Shaw (eds.): *The Biopsychology of Development.* New York, Academic Press, pp. 515–529, 1971.

Engel, G. Attachment behavior, object relations and the dynamic-economic points of view. *Int. J. Psychoanal.,* 52:183–196, 1971.

Engel, G., and Reichsman, F. Spontaneous and experimentally induced depressions in an infant with a gastric fistula. *J. Am. Psychoanal. Assoc.,* 4:428–456, 1956.

Freud, A. Discussion of Dr. Bowlby's paper. *Psychoanal. Study Child,* 15:53–62, 1960.

Freud, A. *Normality and Pathology in Childhood.* New York, International Universities Press, 1965.

Freud, S. (1917) *Mourning and Melancholia, standard ed.* London, Hogarth Press, pp. 237–260, 1957.

Frommer, E. A. Depressive illness in childhood. Recent developments in affective disorders. *Br. J. Psychiatry,* Special Pub. #2:117–136, 1968.

Gero, G. The construction of depression. *Int. J. Psychoanal.,* 17:423–461, 1936.

Gewirtz, J. L. Attachment and dependence: Some strategies and tactics in the selection and use of indices for those concepts, in communication and affect. T. Alloway, L. Krames, P. Pliner (eds.): New York, Academic Press, 1973.

Goldfarb, W. Infant rearing and problem behavior. *Am. J. Orthopsychiatry,* 13:249–265, 1943.

Hill, O. W. Child bereavement and adult psychiatric disturbance. *J. Psychosom. Res.,* 16:357–360, 1972.

Hinde, R. A., and Spencer-Booth, Y. Effects of brief separation from mother on rhesus monkeys. *Science,* 173:111–118, 1971.

Jacobson, E. On normal and pathological moods. *Psychoanal. Study Child,* 12:73–113, 1957.

Jacobson, E. *Acting Out and the Urge to Betray in Paranoid Patients in Depression.* New York, International Universities Press, 1971.

Jarvis, V. Loneliness and compulsion. *J. Am. Psychoanal. Assoc.,* 13:122–158, 1965.

Kasanin, J. The affective psychoses in children. *Am. J. Psychiatry,* 10:897–924, 1931.

Kaufman, I. Three basic sources for pre-delinquent character. *Nerv. Child,* 11:12–15, 1955.

Kaufman, I. C., and Rosenblum, L. A. The reaction to separation in infant monkeys: Anaclitic depression and conservation-withdrawal. *Psychosom. Med.,* 29:648–675, 1967.

Kaufman, I., Durkin, H., Jr., Frank, T., et al. Delineation of two diagnostic groups among juvenile delinquents: The schizophrenic and the impulse-ridden character disorder. *J. Am. Acad. Child Psychiatry,* 2:292–318, 1963.

Klein, M. (1948) *Contributions to Psycho-analysis 1921–1945.* New York, McGraw-Hill, 1964.

Kohut, H. *The Analysis of the Self.* New York, International Universities Press, 1971.

Koran, L. M. The reliability of clinical methods, data and judgments. *N. Engl. J. Med.,* 293:642–646, 1975.

Levin, S. The psychoanalysis of shame. *Int. J. Psychoanal.,* 52:355–362, 1971.

Levy, D. Primary affect hunger. *Am. J. Psychiatry,* 94:643–652, 1937.

Lopez, Ibor J. J. Masked depression. *Br. J. Psychiatry,* 120:245–258, 1972.

Mahler, M. S. On sadness and grief in infancy and childhood. *Psychoanal. Study Child,* 16:332–354, 1961.

Mahler, M. S. Notes on the development of basic moods. In R. Loewenstein, L. Newman, M. Schur, and A. Solnit (eds.): *Psychoanalysis—A General Psychology.* New York, International Universities Press, pp. 152–168, 1966.

Main, A. M. Idealization and disillusion in adolescence. In H. S. Klein (ed.): *Sexuality and Aggression in Maturation: New Facets.* London, Bailliere, Tindall and Cassell, pp. 14–21, 1971.

Malmquist, C. P. Depressions in childhood and adolescence. I. *N. Engl. J. Med.,* 284:887–893, 1971*a*.

Malmquist, C. P. Depressions in childhood and adolescence. II. *N. Engl. J. Med.,* 284:955–961, 1971*b*.

Malmquist, C. P. Depression in childhood. In F. F. Flach and S. Draghi (eds.): *Comprehensive Textbook of Depression.* New York, John Wiley & Sons, 1975.

McConville, B. J., Boag, L. C., and Purohit, A. P. Three types of childhood depression. *Can. Psychiatr. Assoc. J.,* 18:133–138, 1973.

Miller, J. Children's reactions to parent's death. *J. Am. Psychoanal. Assoc.,* 19:697–719, 1971.

Perspective on Human Deprivation. Washington, D. C., U.S. D. H. E. W., 1968.

Poznaski, E., and Zrull, J. P. Childhood depression. *Arch. Gen. Psychiatry,* 23:8–15, 1970.

Rado, S. The problem of melancholia. *Int. J. Psychoanal.,* 9:420–438, 1928.

Reich, A. Pathologic forms of self-esteem regulation. *Psychoanal. Study Child,* 15:215–232, 1960.

Rie, H. E. Depression in childhood: A survey of some pertinent contributions. *J. Am. Acad. Child Psychiatry,* 5:653–685, 1966.

Rochlin, G. The dread of abandonment. *Psychoanal. Study Child,* 16:451–470, 1961.

Rochlin, G. *Loss and Restitution, Grief and Its Discontents.* Boston, Little, Brown and Co., pp. 121–164, 1965.

Rutter, M. *Maternal Deprivation Reassessed.* Baltimore, Penguin Books, 1972.

Sandler, J., and Joffe, W. G. Notes on childhood depression. *Int. J. Psychoanal.,* 46:88–96, 1965.

Schafer, R. The loving and beloved superego in Freud's structural theory. *Psychoanal. Study Child,* 15:163–188, 1960.

Sperling, M. Equivalents of depression in children. *J. Hillside Hosp.,* 8:138–148, 1959.

Spitz, R. Anaclitic depression. *Psychoanal. Study Child,* 2:113–117, 1946.

Suomi, S. J., and Harlow, H. F. Social rehabilitation of isolate-reared monkeys. *Dev. Psychol.,* 6:487–496, 1972.

Symonds, M. The depressions in childhood and adolescence. *Am. J. Psychoanal.,* 28:189–195, 1968.

Winnicott, D. W. (1954) *The Depressive Position in Normal Emotional Development, Collected Papers.* New York, Basic Books, pp. 262–277, 1958.

Wolfenstein, M. How is mourning possible? *Psychoanal. Study Child,* 21:93–126, 1966.

Wooton, B. *Social Science and Social Pathology.* London, Allen and Unwin, 1959.

Young, L. D. Suomi, S. S., Harlow, H. F., and McKinney, W. T. Early stress and later response to separation in rhesus monkeys. *Am. J. Psychiatry,* 130:400–405, 1973.

Discussion of Dr. Malmquist's Chapter:

Childhood Depression: A Clinical and Behavioral Perspective

1. E. James Anthony

Eliot Division of Child Psychiatry, Washington University School of Medicine, St. Louis, Missouri 63130

I have had the opportunity in the past to listen to Dr. Malmquist, and he presents this whole field extremely well. I will comment on one or two things that he said in his chapter or might have said in the past.

First, there is no doubt that there has been a shift in the way we look at children. As you know, psychopathology of childhood, except brain damage and mental retardation, was not evident before the turn of the century. Before the 20th century, people were simply unaware of childhood as an entity, unaware of children as responsibly active individuals in their own right. However, today we are almost obsessed with the total sexual, moral, and physical aspects of childhood. Dr. Malmquist has indicated that children were almost unnoticed—not unloved, but unnoticed as an entity—before this century.

Another point Dr. Malmquist has raised is how our child-rearing practices have been so radically altered from those of previous centuries to the extent that we are beginning to see things in children we have never seen before. Since about 1909 we have viewed children as very responsive, with rich lives, rich ways of looking at the world, and rich ways of experiencing things. Previously, nobody thought of children in these ways. Hence, the climate for recognizing depression in childhood came into being at the beginning of this century, and we are just now able to see and recognize it.

However, as Dr. Malmquist mentioned, once one begins to see something such as childhood depression, one may see it everywhere. We are now calling many things depression, which in the past we did not call depression, and I think we may go over the top and label everything depression. When Leo

Kanner first found autism he said that nobody else could see or recognize it. Nobody had seen it. But once he had seen it, his secretaries could diagnose it in the waiting room.

Another point that Dr. Malmquist raised was the question of the family, and to what extent both culture and the family influence the expression of depression. In our St. Louis sample we divided families into those we called closed families and those that were open-minded. Closed families had little capacity for recognizing affects, dealing with affects, or talking about affects in any significant way. In contrast, in open families affects were in the forefront, so that children were exposed to a constant discussion of feelings. Consequently, in open families feelings could be talked about, expressed, and labeled. In one of the international study groups I participate in, I have observed that the differences in the ways affects are handled within families and within cultures in various parts of the world are quite marked.

Next, I would like to discuss the antecedents of depression and depression proneness. Earlier I mentioned our looking for factors that might lead to proneness for depression. We have now followed many children in our manic-depressive series, and some children have shown what we diagnose as a depressive proclivity, or very early tendency to show depression. It may be evident not in the whole family but in only one of five children, and we then label that particular child at risk. We examine him from the standpoint of his vulnerability or risk and then follow him and make predictions about him.

So far there have been six breakdowns in adolescents (after age 17) in our study. In this age group the breakdowns are not psychotic depressions. However, these children are depressed and they talk about their depressions openly. They also have suicidal wishes and ideas. They have bad self-concepts and feel a loss of pleasure, but they are not psychotic in any way. We have not yet seen in our manic-depressive group any adolescent who has become psychotic. We call their crises breakdowns because we have no other name for them. Earlier on, these children showed a variety of interesting symptoms that again one can understand only as depressive equivalents. Many were difficult babies who became difficult children, who became difficult adolescents and then seemed rather suddenly to become depressed young people.

In relation to what Leon Cytryn mentioned about fantasies and what Dr. Malmquist mentioned about dreams, I had a similar experience I would like to share. I worked with a child named Michael who was very displeased and dissatisfied with himself. Later he was rather reluctant to be with other children and became somewhat withdrawn. There came a moment when he was 9 or 10, when suddenly, after being completely withdrawn and making no contact with his doctor, he said to his doctor, "You know, I have a dream that keeps coming up all the time. Ever since I have been little it has come up."

Before going further into his dream let me supply a few details about this boy. He had been a love child of the mother. She had been deserted while she was pregnant. She brought him up for 5 years and then she remarried and had six children. Suddenly he was introduced to a real family after having lived with his mother alone. In reporting his dream, Michael said, "In the dream I have money, a lot of money, and I lose my money. Well, I don't lose it but I give it to my mother for her to keep, and then when I ask her for it because I want to buy something for myself she tells me that she has already given it to somebody else, that she has given it to my brothers and sisters, and they have spent it, and when I tell my parents they say that there's nothing they can do about it. And this dream comes up over and over." He said he had this dream almost every month. Once he related that dream and cried, the depression began to become very obvious. Nobody had mentioned the word depression before, but when we looked back we could see that he was struggling with depressive affect most of the time, and after he related his dream, it became manifest.

Let me cite one other example. An 8-year-old boy felt a great deal of anger but was unable to express or show it. At times he resembled a caricature of a depressed person but said he was not very depressed. One day he admitted that he was afraid his father might die and had dreams about his father dying. He soon became quite uncooperative and withdrawn. Then, all of a sudden, his father died. After the death of his father he was able to open up and talk about the impact of his father's death. He now was grievously depressed—he cried most of the time.

When he returned to school his teachers wanted to expel him because his behavior had deteriorated terribly; he felt badly about the possibility of being expelled. At his next therapy session he said, "I can't find any images of my father in my mind. He's so far away from me. I'm sad. I feel empty." At the following session he came in with very dirty hands and said, "This is how I used to be. I'm sad all the time." The therapist said, "Do you mean you are sad since your father died?" "No, no, no. Much, much years before he died. I'm the same all the time. I really don't know when I first became sad." The therapist then asked, "Could you tell me when you thought you became sad?" He said, "I think I was sad when I was about 2 years old, but you know why? I think it was when my sister was born." During the next session he was silent, sad, depressed, slow in his mental activity, couldn't cope, and he became worse. Eventually we had to hospitalize him. But the interesting thing is that the depression was latent until the loss of his father, and then suddenly he became quite depressed and traced his depression, not to the father's death, which was pretty rough, but instead to his early life. In fact, he had good reason to be sad because his mother didn't care much for him, and he had felt neglected in the past. The point I would like to make is that it is sometimes difficult to identify depression in children unless cases are followed carefully for extended periods.

2. Leon Cytryn

Unit on Childhood Mental Illness, Adult Psychiatry Branch, National Institutes of Health, Bethesda, Maryland 20014

I would like to address myself first to the chapter of Drs. Kovacs and Beck. Many years ago while searching for a way of rating children, Dr. McKnew and I began by using adult rating scales as a model. We found that this approach led to many pitfalls. I would like to elaborate only one of those, which seems most pertinent since it concerns the self-rating of depressed children. We started simply with a number of cards, each carrying a statement describing a specific mood state. The statements ranged from "I am always very happy" through "I am always very sad," with a great number of mood states sandwiched in between. We then presented the cards to the child asking him to select one card that best represented his feelings. Much to our dismay, the choices of the children were absolutely inconsistent with the clinical picture. Several children who were suicidal, with a history of sad affect, psychomotor retardation, profound hopelessness, social withdrawal, and other depressive symptoms of long duration chose cards such as "I am always happy" or "I am never sad."

In trying to explain this curious response, we thought of several reasons. Most of the depressed children we studied in the past came from the most deprived socioeconomic strata of our population. As a result, they were very unsophisticated in expressing their feelings verbally. Perhaps such a method would be more useful in more sophisticated middle-class children. Another reason for our failure to elicit appropriate self-rating may be related to the age of the children (6 to 12 years). The discrepancy between the child's mood state and his self-rating may decrease with advancing age.

I have sensed a great deal of skepticism about the existence of a clinical entity that may appropriately be called "childhood depression." Some of this skepticism is related to the diverse and manifold phenomena subsumed under this heading by various investigators. Of course, a legitimate concern is that such diversity may preclude the precise delineation of the concept and invite the danger of using the diagnosis of childhood depression loosely as a clinical wastebasket, on par with the most ludicrous diagnostic category in child psychiatry, namely, "the atypical child." I fully agree that we should try to clarify our thinking about the various facets of childhood depression, such as its etiology (McKnew and Cytryn, 1973), course (Cytryn and McKnew, 1972), outcome, response to treatment (McKnew and Cytryn, 1975), and above all, how it differs from other more traditional childhood diagnoses (Cytryn and

McKnew, 1972). The efforts of our own research group, and those of others, some of whom, like Drs. Anthony (1967) and Malmquist (1971a,b), are contributors to this volume, have made some progress in this direction, but obviously much more basic research and conceptualization are needed. On the other hand, is it correct to disregard a clinical phenomenon simply because we do not fully understand it? Such an attitude would be inconsistent with the medical history of most diseases, physical or psychiatric, which were often observed, described, and treated long before all their aspects were well understood.

We should also keep in mind that awareness of the existence of childhood depression is of very recent vintage, and its full understanding will require much work. As happened in the history of many other ideas that lay dormant awaiting their time, there is a sudden awareness of childhood depression as a clinical entity, all over the world, among people of various origins and cultures and diverse professional backgrounds. Obviously, such awareness must be buttressed by scientific proof, which as of now is still lacking.

Permit me to digress for a moment and delve into the history of the parent disease, namely, adult depression. It is probably the oldest disease known to mankind and accorded legitimacy and recognition by all since at least the times of Hippocrates, and yet a few thousand years later controversy still rages about practically every aspect of this disease (Grinker et al., 1961). Such basic concepts as endogenous versus exogenous, neurotic versus psychotic, and acquired versus genetic are still not fully understood. The modern division into unipolar and bipolar illness is already being diluted by subdivisions into several subtypes, the interrelationship of which is quite unclear. To add to the confusion, what about the various subdivisions with high or low urinary 3-methoxy-4-hydroxy phenylethylene glycol (MHPG), a variety of enzyme levels, and electrolyte, steroid, catecholamine, or indolamine disturbances? Mention should also be made of schizoaffective disorders and depressive character and their relationship to other depressive illnesses. Yet despite our lack of perfect understanding, nobody suggests the abolition of the concept of adult depression and its replacement with "dysphoria" or "unhedonia." Quite to the contrary, millions of people yearly are being diagnosed as depressed (often correctly) and treated (often successfully) despite controversial questions.

I suggest that we accord the fledgling childhood depression a similar treatment and approach it with an open mind and patience, rather than dismiss it as an artifact because of its lack of complete clarity as of now.

What has to be overcome is the basic reluctance of many adults, both professionals and nonprofessionals, to admit to the possibility that a child suffers from a depressive illness. Although all people agree to the existence of sadness in children, most consider it to be a transitory phenomenon rather than a chronic, pervasive feature of their personality. I believe that this reluctance on the part of adults leads to an often blatant disregard of long-standing hopelessness, depressive mood, psychomotor retardation, and suicidal ideation even in children whose depressive illness is overt rather than masked. Often such children are shunted into our ossified, imprecise existing diagnostic categories and said to have "withdrawal reaction," "runaway reaction," or "adjustment reaction."

I would like to mention a situation in which the training and attitude of psychiatrists rather than the actual clinical picture determined the diagnosis of the patients. The Cross-National Project for the Study of the Diagnosis of Mental Disorders in the United States and United Kingdom (Gurland et al., 1972) investigated the cross-national differences reported in the public mental hospital statistics on admission rates of schizophrenics (preponderant in the United States) and those with manic-depressive disorders (preponderant in the United Kingdom). This ingenious study clearly revealed that the intriguing cross-national differences are attributable not to a real difference in the prevalence of the two illnesses but rather to the background and diagnostic habits of American and British psychiatrists, the former being more inclined to diagnose schizophrenia, whereas the latter prefer the manic-depressive label.

This study as well as the International Pilot Study of Schizophrenia (Sartorius et al., 1974) also points to some methodologic strategies useful in the study of psychiatric illness lacking diagnostic precision and consensus when examined by people with diverse professional backgrounds. Some of those strategies have been mentioned elsewhere in this volume as potentially useful in the study of childhood depression: namely (1) use of structured interviews to ensure uniform eliciting of information; (2) use of standardized ratings on items of psychopathology defined in straightforward operational language; (3) collaboration of several research teams, which all use the agreed upon diagnostic methods; and (4) close collaboration among the various investigators, which would include comparison of videotaped interviews and ongoing communication to deal with and clarify diagnostic differences whenever they arise.

Our group is presently conducting a double-blind study of (1) the offspring of depressed adults and (2) the offspring of two control groups. We use both "blind" and "naive" interviewers and raters. We hope that when this study is completed (hopefully to be followed by similar studies by other investigators) we will be in a better position to have scientific proof for or against the existence of childhood depression as a clinical entity.

I would like to make a few comments about the concept of masked depression in children, which seems to face the stiffest opposition, reminding us of the controversy over the concept of depressive equivalents in adults. Our team stumbled on this diagnostic concept by happenstance. When we examined children with overt unequivocal depressive symptoms, our examination included a lengthy exploration of their fantasy life as is customary in child psychiatry. We found that these fantasies have a common leitmotif, namely, something unpleasant and harmful happening to the main character.

Unlike depressed adults, depressed children seldom see themselves as the dramatis personae of their fantasies but substitute an animal, cartoon character, or even an inanimate object. The things that happened in these fantasies ranged from being trapped, frustrated, exploited, or ridiculed to being killed, injured, and committing suicide. When we explored the fantasies of children with overt anxiety reactions, we found similar themes but also a fundamental difference. In the anxious children, there was usually a threat of something unpleasant and harmful happening to the main character. The threat, however, was never actually carried to its tragic conclusion. Someone pursued the hero of the fantasy, but he was able to get away—he was falling down a cliff but woke up before he hit the ground, etc. This was in contrast to the fantasies of depressed children, in which the unpleasant, harmful, or tragic conclusion actually occurred.

When we examined many children who had no overt depressive symptomatology but rather presented with behavior problems, aggression or delinquency, psychosomatic illness, school phobia, and many other diverse clinical pictures, we were intrigued by finding in some of these children the same kind of fantasy pervaded by hopelessness and helplessness as found previously in overtly depressed children. When we scrutinized these children, their parents, and their teachers more closely, we invariably found a history of intermittent periods of overtly depressive verbal and nonverbal symptomatology lasting for several days, weeks, or even months. Thus, we postulated that masked depressive reactions in children include two phenomena: (1) the presence of predominantly depressive fantasy; and (2) the presence of definite, verified periods of overt depressive symptomatology.

After having postulated the concept of masked depression in children, previously described independently by Glaser (1967), we still share the uncertainty expressed by some contributors to this volume about the clinical specificity of this diagnostic category and especially its relationship to overt depressive illness in children. In the last 2 years we had an opportunity to examine these questions in the framework of a study of children and grandchildren of manic-depressive patients, conducted by our team in the Unit on Childhood Mental Illness of the NIMH, Adult Psychiatry Branch (McKnew et al., 1976). When we examined the children for the first time, we found many of them presenting a very depressive fantasy but no overt depressive symptomatology. In our assessment of these first interviews, despite our conviction that masked depression is a viable clinical entity, we decided for reasons of research clarity to rate those children as presenting no significant psychopathology. Much to our surprise, when these children were interviewed the second time, 4 months later (always by a different interviewer), most of them had overt depression. This finding, which we continue to pursue, indicates that what we call masked depressive reaction may very well be related to childhood depression and should not be lightly dismissed as a clinical nonentity without further exploration.

Finally, only future research will clarify the controversial issue of the relationship between adult and childhood depression. There are several possibilities:

1. Both adult and childhood depressions are part of a spectrum of depressive disorders, the expression and the incidence of which are dependent on the given level of personality development.

2. Childhood depression leads to or predisposes toward depression in later life.

3. Despite clinical similarities, childhood and adult depressions, because of their disparity in etiology and course, can best be thought of as representing separate, independent entities.

REFERENCES

Anthony, E. J. Psychoneurotic disorders. In A. M. Freedman and H. G. Kaplan (eds.): *Comprehensive Textbook of Psychiatry*. Baltimore, Williams & Wilkins Co., pp. 1387–1406, 1967.

Cytryn, L., and McKnew, D. H., Jr. Proposed classification of childhood depression. *Am. J. Psychiatry,* 129:149–155, 1972.

Glaser, K. Masked depression in children and adolescents. *Am. J. Psychother.,* 21:565–574, 1967.

Grinker, R. R., Miller, J., Sabshin, M., Nunn, R., and Nunnally, J. C. *The Phenomena of Depressions*. New York, Harper & Row, 1961.

Gurland, B. J., Fleiss, J. L., Barrett, J. E., Jr., Sharpe, L., and Simon, R. J. The mislabeling of depressed patients in New York State hospitals. In J. Zubin and F. A. Freyhan (eds.): *Disorders of Mood*. Baltimore, Johns Hopkins University Press, pp. 17–31, 1972.

Malmquist, C. P. Depressions in childhood and adolescence. I. *N. Engl. J. Med.,* 284:887–893, 1971a.

Malmquist, C. P. Depressions in childhood and adolescence. II. *N. Engl. J. Med.,* 284:955–961, 1971b.

McKnew, D. H., Jr., and Cytryn, L. Historical background in children with affective disorders. *Am. J. Psychiatry,* 130:11, 1973.

McKnew, D. H., Jr., and Cytryn, L. Detection and treatment of childhood depression. Paper read at the annual meeting of the American Psychiatric Association, Anaheim, California, May 7, 1975.

McKnew, D. H., Jr., Cytryn, L., Efron, A., Gershon, E. S., and Bunney, W. E., Jr. Offspring of manic-depressive patients. Paper read at the annual meeting of the American Psychiatric Association, Miami, Florida, May 12, 1976.

Sartorius, N., Shapiro, R., and Jablensky, A. The International Pilot Study of Schizophrenia. *Schizophrenia Bull.,* 11:21–34, 1974.

Depression in Childhood: Diagnosis, Treat-
ment, and Conceptual Models, edited by J. G.
Schulterbrandt and A. Raskin. Raven Press,
New York, 1977.

Definitional and Methodological Issues
Concerning Depressive Illness in Children

Rachel Gittelman-Klein

*Queens College, City University of New York, Flushing, New York, and Child
Development Clinic, Long Island Jewish-Hillside Medical Center,
Glen Oaks, New York 11004*

INTRODUCTION

The term "depression" presents great semantic ambiguity. It has both
vernacular and psychiatric meanings, whose distinct respective connotations
are often obscured. In everyday usage, depression refers to a subjective mood
state exclusively. There is no concern for concomitant alterations of cognition
or competence, such as changes in self-esteem, level of activity, interest, or
shifts in ability to meet usual role expectations. When laymen use the word
depression, they are referring to unhappiness, or misery. This concept of
depression overlaps with that used in descriptive psychiatry but does not
coincide with it.

Although no unanimous psychiatric definition of depression exists, the
concept of adult depression carries a twofold clinical connotation. On the one
hand, it refers to a state, trait, or symptom, which may occur in varying
severity as a secondary complication in a diversity of mental or physical
disorders such as phobias, schizophrenia, organic mental syndromes, and
other conditions. In such cases, one would describe the patients as depressed
but not necessarily as suffering from a depressive illness. On the other hand,
depression is a pathological clinical entity that regularly implies a reduction in
hedonic level, loss of interest, and a diminution in one's sense of competence,
all in the context of a dysphoric state or psychic pain. This state is accompanied by a number of other symptoms that have been given differing emphases
by various investigators. Some have stressed loss of self-esteem, others guilt,
others retardation of mental activity, and yet others alterations of basic
biological functions (e.g., sleeping, eating, elimination) as important aspects of
depressive illness. Although disagreements exist concerning whether the
mood or cognitive attitudinal symptoms are primary or secondary in adult

depressive illness, their stipulation enables objective, empirical determination of the merits of the various schemas.

The history of classification of adult mood disorders can be used as a model for the study of other psychiatric disorders of childhood or adulthood. A confluence of data accumulated through the study of the disorders' natural course, response to pharmacologic intervention, and genetics has made disorders of mood the best-understood psychiatric states with clear therapeutic and prognostic implications.

Other adult dysphoric states, sometimes referred to as "atypical depressions" or "minor mood disorders," are more complex than unhappiness, yet do not conform clearly to the criteria of the phasic pathological clinical syndromes. Many clinical aspects, such as source or treatment response, of the "atypical" mood disorders are still relatively unknown. Despite the existence of poorly understood depressive states, relatively homogeneous clinical subgroups have been identified within the broad category of mood disorders.

The study of childhood depression has not met, as yet, as happy a scientific fate as the study of adult disorders.

DEFINITIONAL PROBLEMS

Kovacs and Beck *(this volume)* have provided a lucid comprehensive review of the clinical descriptions of samples of "depressed" children.

A critical perusal of the extensive literature on depression in children reveals a failure to provide a well-defined clinical picture common to children said to suffer from depression. There is as yet no single substantiated syndromal description of childhood depression.

The diagnosis in childhood has been bedevilled by serious definitional problems. It has been used to encompass a variety of affect states such as unhappiness, grief, disappointment, demoralization, and helplessness to name but a few. Only one clinical description of childhood depression (Anthony, 1967) includes diminished capacity for self-enjoyment as part of the condition. The proposed classification of childhood disorders in the Group for the Advancement of Psychiatry (GAP) report (1966), whose authors made a serious effort to provide comprehensive clinical diagnoses in pediatric psychiatry, fails as well to provide rules or even guidelines toward a definition of depression in children. The report states, "Depression in children and even in adolescents may be manifested in ways somewhat different from those manifested by adults. These include eating and sleeping disturbances, hyperactivity, and other patterns. The picture of depression may be much more clear and marked, particularly when precipitated by an actual, threatened, or symbolic loss of a parent or parent substitute. Loss of self-esteem, feelings of self-depreciation, guilt, and ambivalence toward the loved person may be present in older children, as in adults. However, psychomotor retardation is ordinarily less marked than in adults, and, except in young infants, the same is true of some of the other biologic signs of depression." The above diagnosis of psychoneurotic depression is confusingly defined by specifying symptoms that do *not* rule out the condition; it does not stipulate inclusion or exclusion criteria, thus ensuring diagnostic chaos.

To complicate matters further, depression in children is often inferred from the presence of disparate behaviors such as aggression, hyperactivity, enuresis, sleeping and eating disturbances, and somatic complaints, sometimes in the absence of clear mood changes or dysphoria. These behavior patterns, labeled "masked depressions," or "depressive equivalents," are construed to be markers for an underlying depressive disorder that is interpreted to account for a multitude of behavior problems, even though depression itself is not clearly manifest. There is no compelling logic to the above view. As likely a hypothesis is that children who are in conflict with their environment become morose, developing secondary depressive symptomatology. It is not self-evident that hyperactive and acting-out behaviors regularly represent defenses against depression. It is equally likely that hyperactive children develop negative attitudes toward themselves and a pessimistic view of their potential for reaping satisfaction from their interpersonal interactions as a consequence of the chronic lack of positive feedback that has characterized their experiences. It is now widely argued that poor self-esteem is a common complication in hyperactive youngsters. Similarly, a phobic child may become dejected because of objective appreciation of his shortcomings, which set him apart from his peers and from his previous symptom-free functioning. The postulation of an underlying depressive disorder in a variety of pediatric behavior disorders is hardly indispensable to our understanding of these disorders. Alternate clinical interpretations are possible which do not rely on the concept of a primary pathological mood state.

The field of childhood depression is in the singular position of having an unspecified, undocumented disorder for which numerous equivalents are postulated.

Only three studies were found that specify minimum operational criteria for a diagnosis of depression in children (Ling et al., 1970; Rideau, 1971; Weinberg et al., 1973). In one of these (Ling et al., 1970), the determination for depression was made retrospectively. In the other two outstanding studies, the data sources and the information domain sampled are unknown; it is unexplained whether reliance was placed on the child's self-report, on the parent's, on the school's, on direct observations, or whether judgments were derived from a combination of these sources. No information concerning reliability is offered.

It seems fair to state that no clinical syndrome of depression has been identified in children. The outstanding exception is Bowlby's (1969) description of young children separated from their parenting figures. However, it may be argued that these children are viewed better as experiencing mourning rather than a primary dysphoric disorder. Cytryn and McKnew (1972) have also reported on a depressive syndrome that may take acute or chronic forms. However, all the children developed the syndrome in the context of marked environmental adversity, and the children improved within days of removal from home, which raises questions regarding the degree to which the childhood symptomatology corresponds to adult depressive illness that is not typically related to external events and does not respond to simple environmental manipulation. In a recent review, Conners (1976) emphasized that similar mood disorders present with different signs and symptoms in children and adults because of the former's immature cognitive processes, personality structure, etc. Although possibly correct, this postulation is untestable without knowledge of the pathophysiology of depression. Such information would enable determination of the variety of manifest symptoms associated with the underlying disorder. This level of understanding is not likely to be forthcoming in the near future.

In the meantime, grouping widely disparate syndromes on the basis of an inferred underlying shared primary dysfunction is probably counterproductive. This view, similar to that formulated for schizophrenia by Bleuler, led to the abandonment of the kraepelinian descriptive approach and to the unjustified proliferation of the diagnosis, virtually removing from the category much of its predictive validity with regard to outcome—better not let history repeat itself. This is not to say that there is no merit in postulating different mood regulatory processes in children and adults. It is quite conceivable that central hedonic receptors differ with age. Children display more adient approach behavior than adults do. In addition, their natural or usual mood is more elevated, joyful, and more labile than that of adults. Children typically feel happy whereas grown-ups do not—the mood state of adults is neutral. Therefore, it seems that the observations made on normal children would lead to the postulation of dissimilar affective regulators among immature and mature individuals, rather than to the postulation of identical mood regulation; children and adults differing only with regard to the superficial, manifest concomitants of various mood states. If it is indeed correct that the central regulatory mechanisms of normal mood differ in early versus later life, it is unlikely that pathological dysregulations of these processes follow similar patterns across all ages.

Rutter and Graham (1968) compared psychiatric clinical interview ratings given blindly to normal children and young psychiatric patients. Ratings of depression were significantly greater among the patients than among the normals. However, they were not different among the three clinical groups: neurotic, antisocial, and mixed diagnoses. This finding suggests that what is labeled depression in children occurs across all diagnostic groups and does not represent a separate, discrete pathological entity. This concept of depression is akin to the one in adult psychiatry wherein depressive symptomatology may be superimposed on a variety of disabilities without representing a well-defined psychiatric entity. We are then dealing with depressive traits rather than a mood disorder.

METHODOLOGICAL ISSUES

Some basic requirements must be met in an attempt to derive diagnostic clarity: the most crucial and problematic is the stipulation of necessary and sufficient clinical characteristics for the diagnosis of childhood depression; the life circumstances associated with the clinical condition need to be documented; the child's previous psychosocial history requires investigation; the reliability of both the clinical judgments and evaluations of the child's environment are necessary; finally, the validity of the condition must be established.

Clinical Criteria

Given the basic necessity for providing objective, reliable criteria for a current diagnosis of depression in children, how does one begin to differentiate among the various affects associated with mental anguish or psychic pain? What distinction can be made among unhappiness, helplessness, disappointment, grief, demoralization, and pathological dysphoria—the emotional conditions most frequently subsumed under the rubric of depression? Reliance on a sad demeanor as a classificatory criterion for depression is fraught with problems. As Werry (1976) has pointed out, if the mere presence of dysphoric symptoms forms a sufficient basis for a diagnosis of childhood depression, we run the danger of broadening the category to such a point as to render it meaningless. The pitfalls inherent in using sad mood as a cardinal diagnostic criterion have been reviewed pointedly by Graham (1974). Since sad affect is found in many different psychiatric and nonpsychiatric disorders, it is easy to accept that one should not rely strongly on the presence of a sad appearance for a diagnosis of depression. But even dramatic symptoms, such as suicide ideation or suicidal attempts, can be misleading regarding their contribution to the diagnosis of depression. Reports dealing with suicide among children and young adolescents, although not unanimous, are astonishing in their consistency: in the majority of children, suicide ideation and attempts are not associated with concurrent clinical depressions (Bakwin, 1957; Fisher, 1971; Koski, 1971; Tadić et al., 1971; Shaffer, 1974).

The challenge, then, is to identify cardinal symptoms with construct validity for depression which will provide a heuristic framework for the study of the disorder in children.

A useful approach might be to identify children who have a pervasive and autonomous loss of hedonic experience. These children would be defined by their lack of age-appropriate response to usually pleasurable activities in a variety of settings. A diminished ability to experience pleasure would have to be observed and reported by the significant adults in the child's life. In essence, depressed children, as Anthony (1967) has put it, cannot be cheered up. Therefore, shifts in the child's immediate environment do not result in relatively prompt mood amelioration.

From the current reports, such children are likely to be rare, and perhaps nonexistent in preschool ages, as suggested by the observed prevalence of 1 to 2 per 1,000 in the Isle of Wight survey (Rutter, Tizard, and Whitmore, 1970) and by a report of seven endogenous depressives (criteria unspecified) among 1,600 Turkish psychiatric patients between the ages of 3 and 16 (Cebiroglu, Sumer, and Polvan, 1971). In Rutter et al.'s report, the two pure depressive states were among older children; the Turkish group does not indicate whether the seven cases of endogenous depression were restricted to the older group or were distributed throughout the age range.

Children likely to be identified in relatively large numbers are those whose affective responses are variable. Although they may display a lack of joyful responsivity in certain settings, they can enjoy themselves in other situations and can exhibit mood elevation when their external circumstances are altered. Given this large undifferentiated heterogeneous group, uniform only with regard to the presence of fluctuating dysphoria, at least two further clinical assessments of current functioning are called for: (1) identification of children with concurrent behavior problems; and (2) identification of children with unsatisfactory home environments (these two conditions are not mutually exclusive).

Care should be taken to identify clearly children with other concomitant behavior or emotional disorders to avoid the almost general logical pitfall of attributing a primary role to the depressive symptomatology and interpreting other deviance as secondary complications of an underlying mood disorder.

This initial approach would identify four subgroups of "depressed" children: (1) those with pervasive endogenous depressive disorders, (2) children with situational dysphorias, and (3) and (4) two more groups of children with the above mood disorders accompanied by other behavioral problems. Children with behavior problems whose mood state does not meet the criteria for depression would be omitted. Therefore, it is suggested that "depressive equivalents," which are the products of dubious psychodynamic theoretical inferences, not be included in this group of conditions until empirical data demonstrate relationships among the behaviors masking depression and manifest depressive disorders.

For purposes of quantifying the concept of decreased hedonic response, different approaches are necessary at different developmental levels. Obviously, the younger the child, the less the reliance on interview and the greater the reliance on controlled observation. Clinical instrument development is sorely lacking in child psychiatry. An initial attempt to meet this need has been made by the Psychopharmacology Research Branch of the NIMH, which has published a battery of clinical rating forms to ensure uniformity of clinical data obtained in psychopharmacologic studies of children (ECDEU, 1973). Only some, unfortunately not all, of the instruments have demonstrated reliability as well as validity for their intended purpose, in this instance, the study of drug effects.

Rutter and Graham (1968) have also devised a psychiatric interview rating form for children. Like the NIMH forms, it was not intended for the identification of mood disorders.

Careful delineation of mood disorders in children is required with different operational criteria for the core dysfunction at several developmental levels (6 to 12 months; 13 to 24 months; 25 months to 3 years, 11 months; 4 to 6 years; up to puberty but not above 12 years). The age of children is limited to 12, even if puberty has not occurred, because many prepubertal youngsters over 12 experience a shift in reference group, in process of identification, and in their role in the family, and they may be more similar to older adolescents than to younger children.

The behavioral domain sampled for these measures cannot be restricted to office or hospital observations of the child. Behaviors in situations in which the child spends significant portions of his time need to be recorded.

The approach developed by Katz and Lyerly (1963) for quantifying reports on patient's behavior by family members can be used as a model in first attempts to meet the effort of obtaining objective information regarding the child's behavior at home. The Teacher Rating Form by Conners (1969) has proved extremely valuable in identifying hyperactive children, as well as in studying drug effects in these children, but the form would probably need elaboration and inclusion of different items relevant to mood states to be useful in the study of depression.

In addition to the presence of dysphoria, other ratings of current clinical status will be required. These include: (1) other mood states such as hostility, anxiety, both generalized and specific, pessimism, and hypomania; (2) attitude, self-esteem, and expressed goals; (3) motor functions such as retardation, mutism, pressure of speech, rigidity; (4) biological functioning, i.e., sleeping, eating (anorexia, overeating, bulimia, weight loss or gain), elimination (enuresis, encopresis, diarrhea, constipation); (5) social functioning with peers, siblings, and adults in and out of school; (6) school performance, including attention and achievement (decrements in academic function should be based on quantitative academic ratings or tests rather than on global impressions that the child is not doing as well); (7) other symptoms, compulsions, obsessions, nervous habits, and conduct problems.

Associated Psychosocial Factors

In the evaluation of childhood depression it seems essential to include an assessment of the adequacy of the child's environment with regard to nutrition, nurturance, opportunity for independent functioning, discipline, rewards, changes in family constellation, and other factors.

The pattern which emerges from the literature is that the vast majority of children beyond infancy who constitute the clinical case material of reports on depression come from homes that grossly fail to meet their emotional and often physical needs. Descriptions of the familial environments of the children read like a compilation of the Brothers Grimm's tales. Therefore, it seems possible to view the children's behavior as a reactive, rather than an organismic, endogenous pathological process. These children have little escape available from their unrewarding environments. They are unhappy. Unhappy, distraught individuals assume multiform behaviors to ward off noxious stimuli, to retaliate, to escape, to find some source of comfort and satisfaction. Perhaps even when the unhappiness is alleviated, the secondary adaptive or defensive behaviors retain functional autonomy. As a result the children's disruptive behavior, which originated during a period of unhappiness, continues and is then interpreted as masking depression since it was originally observed during a dysphoric state.

The regular identification of familial situations likely to engender misery in children might clarify the relationship between mood deterioration and behavior problems. Reliable, valid measures of children's psychosocial milieus need to be devised. Reliability of the assessment of associated events (precipitants, home and school environments) requires well-defined, discrete categories since it has already been demonstrated that global impressions are unreliable (Rutter, Shaffer, and Shepherd, 1973). A salient problem in this area is the construct validity of the ratings. How well do evaluations of the home environment reflect what actually goes on in the home?

Previous History

In addition to concerns of the usual history of the child's rate of development and general adjustment, special attention should be paid to the child's history of response to normal separation experiences, and the history of bereavement or parental separation since a relationship between separation and depression has been postulated (Brown, 1966; Caplan and Douglas, 1969). Results have been contradictory, but it is conceivable that among the larger group of depressed children, those with antecedent significant bereavement may represent a different clinical subgroup with specific treatment and prognostic implications. Further, a history should provide an indication as to whether the child's current status represents one of five possible patterns of illness: (1) development of a depressive disorder in a previously normally functioning child; (2) continuation of a relatively stable chronic condition; (3) exacerbation of an ongoing chronic disorder; (4) recent superimposition of a depressive state in a disturbed child (the type of disturbance being specified); and, finally,

(5) a periodic course of a dysphoric state, superimposed on an unremarkable or disordered pattern of adjustment.

Reliability

Unfortunately, it cannot be assumed that if clinicians believe they understand the meaning of depression in children, they will be likely to agree in their observations and judgments regarding its manifestation. In Rutter and Graham's study of the interrater reliability of a structured psychiatric examination, the two least reliable items were those dealing with affect.

In addition, very low reliability was found in evaluating depressive affect and thought content in different interviews with an interval of 1 to 30 days (mean of 12 days). In this instance, the interrater agreement was extremely low ($r = 0.25$ and 0.04, respectively, for depression and preoccupation with depressive topics). This finding suggests that the child's behaviors used to infer depression are unstable and inconstant. Therefore, the study brings to light pitfalls inherent in procedures that rely on observations made during interviews and on information elicited exclusively from the child for the determination of affective illness in children. The low reliability for ratings of depression is all the more striking since it was obtained by two psychiatrists who had worked together and who had undertaken joint training with the instrument before the reliability study. If easy consensus could be expected, these investigators should be the most likely to obtain it. Their findings underline the necessity for clear diagnostic criteria for depression.

Validity

It is hoped that careful, systematic identification of children with deficits in the capacity for pleasure experiences will yield relatively homogeneous clinical groups. Questions still remain regarding the significance of the disorders identified. Do all or only some, if any, represent variants of adult depressive disorders?

Several approaches can be used to validate the relationship between early childhood and later mood disorders. The two most convincing sources of data for establishing an association between childhood and adult mood disorders are follow-up studies of depressed children into adulthood and prevalence studies of adult depression in the relatives of depressed youngsters. Both methods inevitably require appropriate comparison groups. Some studies have appeared reporting on the frequency of depressive illness in the parents of depressed children. However, the data are almost uninterpretable because of the vagueness of criteria for depression in both the children and their parents, the frequent lack of controls, and the universal lack of blind to the children's diagnoses while making judgments about their relatives. A third avenue in the investigation of genetic factors in childhood depression is that currently used in schizophrenia—the study of offspring of adults with mood disorders. The practical methodological problem in the "high-risk" research model is the requirement for extremely large samples to enable identification of enough individuals who eventually develop the disorder under study (in this instance, depression).

Several long-term studies have reported on the adult status of young patients. Some have contrasted the outcome of children who had "depressive" symptoms to those without such a history. However, no systematic attempt to identify depressive symptomatology specifically was made originally when the children were evaluated, and it is quite conceivable that a large number of false-negative cases with regard to depression in early years were included, thereby minimizing the likelihood of finding meaningful relationships between early history and later functioning. A further difficulty in conducting follow-ups among young depressives is that long lag may occur between episodes. Even if children suffering from depression were likely to become depressed in adulthood, they might not do so until relatively late, such as in their 30s. Therefore, although they yield valuable information, prospective long-term studies are impractical. The most direct, rapid, and economical method for determining the relationship between childhood and adult mood disorders is study of the genetic characteristics of childhood depression. This approach has certainly been useful in another childhood disorder, childhood schizophrenia, where genetic studies failed to reveal an increased prevalence of schizophrenia in the relatives of the children. These findings have led to a skeptical attitude toward the theory that childhood schizophrenia represents an early manifestation of the adult disorder.

Should genetic studies of carefully delineated childhood depression disorders fail to reveal a significant concordance among relatives, then a new term for childhood depression will need to be coined. It is most undesirable to use identical diagnostic descriptive labels for different clinical syndromes, since diagnoses often carry therapeutic and etiologic messages. If depressions in childhood are qualitatively different from those in adulthood, it is unlikely, although not impossible, that antidepressants will contribute to their improvement. Yet, if use of the term childhood depression as a diagnosis persists, there is little doubt that the use of so-called antidepressant compounds will be extended inappropriately to children.

Yet another approach used to investigate diagnostic relationships among disorders is to study their respective responses to treatment. The assumption that two disorders share a common pathophysiological defect if they both respond to the same drug is fraught with pitfalls. Psychiatric drugs have complex, multisystem actions; the inference that identical biochemical processes are responsible for alterations of disparate states is premature given our limited knowledge of drugs' pharmacology.

An example in point is citing the responsiveness of enuresis to imipramine to reinforce the claim that the symptom is a depressive equivalent. There is now evidence that the imipramine effect in enuresis may be owing to the drug's effect on the bladder, or possibly the peripheral nervous system, not to its action on the central nervous system. Although controlled studies of antidepressants should be investigated in childhood depressions, the fact that they may be efficacious is not a crucial test of the association between the childhood and adult disorders. On the other hand, diagnostic subgroups might emerge among depressed children as a result of identifiable consistent differential patterns of drug response.

SUMMARY

The diagnosis of depression in children is ill-defined and refers to a multitude of behavioral symptoms.

Emphasis should be placed on identifying children with demonstrable decreases in their ability to experience pleasure. It is suggested that this characteristic be used as a central clinical criterion for the identification of childhood depression. The most expedient and valid means of determining its relationship to adult depressions is through genetic studies. However, until empirical data are gathered, there is little justification for assuming that unhappy children are miniature versions of adults with mood disorders. Therefore, exception is taken to a statement which appeared in a recent publication on depression that, "For most diagnostic purposes at present, perhaps nothing more is needed than a diagnosis of 'Childhood Depression' indicating its presence" (Malmquist, 1975, p. 89). Rather, the path to follow is that suggested by Prugh et al. (1975), "the only possible approach to a system of classification of disturbed behavior in childhood and adolescence today is a typological one which is primarily descriptive (rather than explanatory) and based on operational definitions" (pp. 265–266).

REFERENCES

Anthony, E. J. Psychiatric disorders of childhood. II: Psychoneurotic, psychophysiological and personality disorders. In: A. M. Freedman and H. G. Kaplan (eds.): *Comprehensive Textbook of Psychiatry*. Baltimore, Williams & Wilkins Co., pp. 1433–1438, 1967.
Bakwin, H. Suicide in children and adolescents. *J. Pediatr.,* 50:749–769, 1957.
Bowlby, J. *Attachment and Loss, Vol. 1.* New York; Basic Books, 1969.
Brown, F. Childhood bereavement and subsequent psychiatric disorder. *Br. J. Psychiatry,* 112:1035–1041, 1966.
Caplan, M. G., and Douglas, V. I. Incidence of parental loss in children with depressed mood. *J. Child Psychol. Psychiatry,* 10:225–232, 1969.
Cebiroglu, R., Sumer, E., and Polvan, O. Etiology and pathogenesis of depression in Turkish children. In A.-L. Annell (ed.): *Depressive States in Childhood and Adolescence.* Stockholm, Almqvist & Wiksell, pp. 133–136, 1971.
Conners, C. K. A teacher rating scale. *Am. J. Psychiatry,* 126:152–156, 1969.

Conners, C. K. Classification and treatment of childhood depression and depressive equivalents. In D. M. Gallant and G. M. Simpson (eds.): *Depression: Behavioral, Biochemical, Diagnostic and Treatment Concepts.* Holliswood, N.Y., Spectrum Publications, pp. 196–199, 1976.

Cytryn, L., and McKnew, D. H. Proposed classification of childhood depression. *Am. J. Psychiatry,* 129:149–155, 1972.

ECDEU [Early Clinical Drug Evaluation Unit] Assessment Battery for Pediatric Psychopharmacology. Washington, D.C., NIMH Psychopharmacology Research Branch, 1973.

Fisher, J. Depressive states and suicidal thoughts in children. In A.-L. Annell (ed.): *Depressive States in Childhood and Adolescence.* Stockholm, Almqvist & Wiksell, pp. 326–328, 1971.

Graham, P. Depression in pre-pubertal children. *Dev. Med. Child Neurol.,* 16:340–349, 1974.

Group for the Advancement of Psychiatry. *A Proposed Classification of Psychopathological Disorders in Children.* New York, Group for the Advancement of Psychiatry, 1966.

Katz, M. M., and Lyerly, S. B. Methods for measuring adjustment and social behavior in the community. I. Rationale, description, discriminative validity and scale development. *Psychol. Rep.,* 13:503–535, 1963.

Koski, M.-L. The suicidal behavior of young adolescents. In A.-L. Annell (ed.): *Depressive States in Childhood and Adolescence.* Stockholm, Almqvist & Wiksell, pp. 329–334, 1971.

Ling, W., Oftedal, G., and Weinberg, W. Depressive illness in childhood presenting as severe headache. *Am. J. Dis. Child.,* 120:122–124, 1970.

Malmquist, C. P. Depression in childhood. In F. F. Flach and S. C. Draghi (eds.): *The Nature and Treatment of Depression.* New York, John Wiley & Sons, pp. 73–98, 1975.

Prugh, D. G., Engel, M., and Morse, W. C. Emotional disturbance in children. In N. Hobbs (ed.): *Issues in the Classification of Children, Vol. 1.* San Francisco, Jossey-Bass Publishers, pp. 261–299, 1975.

Rideau, A. Les états dépressifs du débile profond jeune (Depressive states in profound mental retardation). In A.-L. Annell (ed.): *Depressive States in Childhood and Adolescence.* Stockholm, Almqvist & Wiksell, pp. 126–132, 1971.

Rutter, M., and Graham, P. The reliability and validity of the psychiatric assessment of the child: I. Interview with the child. *Br. J. Psychiatry,* 114:563–579, 1968.

Rutter, M., Shaffer, D., and Shepherd, M. An evaluation of the proposal for a multi-axial classification of child psychiatric disorders. *Psychol. Med,* 3:244–250, 1973.

Rutter, M., Tizard, J., and Whitmore, K. *Education, Health and Behavior.* London, Longman, 1970.

Shaffer, D. Suicide in childhood and early adolescence. *J. Child Psychol. Psychiatry,* 15:275–291, 1974.

Tadić, N., Radulovic-Mihaljević, K., and Antonić, Z. La tentative de suicide comme un symptome de la dépression chez les enfants et les adolescents (Attempted suicide as a sign of depression in children and adolescents). In A.-L. Annell (ed.): *Depressive States in Childhood and Adolescence.* Stockholm, Almqvist & Wiksell, pp. 335–339, 1971.

Weinberg, W. A., Rutman, J., Sullivan, L., Penick, E. C., and Dietz, S. G. Depression in children referred to an educational diagnostic center: Diagnosis and treatment. *J. Pediatr.,* 83:1065–1072, 1973.

Werry, J. Commentary on Conners, C. K., classification and treatment of childhood depression and depressive equivalents. In D. M. Gallant and G. M. Simpson (eds.): *Depression: Behavioral, Biochemical, Diagnostic and Treatment Concepts.* Holliswood, N.Y., Spectrum Publications, pp. 196–199, 1976.

Discussion of Dr. Gittelman-Klein's Chapter:

Definitional and Methodological Issues Concerning Depressive Illness in Children

Monroe M. Lefkowitz

New York State Department of Mental Hygiene, Albany, New York 12229

At this time no statistically reliable or valid measure of depression exists for children. This point was consistently made in Dr. Gittelman's chapter. We have only clinical evaluations and clinical impressions based on appearance and/or samples of behavior of the child obtained during clinical interview, from case materials, or from both.

Clinically, a child is described as depressed if he manifests any of a wide variety of behaviors with some degree of frequency: withdrawal, crying, school failure, aggressions, somatic complaints, avoidance of eye contact, and others. Indeed, almost any behavior aversive enough to prod parents into referring the child for professional help may earn the child a label of "depressed." But, as Dr. Gittelman urges, no criteria for inclusion or exclusion are stipulated for applying this label.

This operation of symptom presentation, referral, and diagnosis raises the broader questions of sampling bias, prevalence of depressive symptoms in clinic versus normal or controlled samples, and epidemiology. In the case of sampling bias, the clinician obviously sees only those children who are referred. But many of the behaviors under consideration are broadly distributed among the general childhood population. The same behavior that seems salient enough to warrant referral for one set of parents may not be so for another. Moreover, the likelihood is great that such saliency will vary with parents' education and socioeconomic status. Theoretically, one would also expect variability for any one child and for groups of children in the manifestation of behaviors classified as depressive. Moreover, if the classification of childhood depression is to have any validity, it is of overriding importance to be able to differentiate this response style, trait, or dimension from transient developmental phenomena visible in normal children.

Leo Kanner (1960) notes that the exaggerated psychopathological significance attached to single behaviors arises from the use of statistics contributed by selected groups of children from child guidance clinics and juvenile courts.

In the general population of children, the occurrence and psychiatric fate of these so-called symptoms are unknown. Dr. Gittelman rightly stresses the need for follow-up studies of a clinical population.

Herbert Quay (1972) states that with respect to the definition of any disorder, the first step is to demonstrate that a constellation of behaviors can be reliably observed in one or more situations that define the disorder. Once a definition such as depressive order is applied to a child, information about etiology and outcome is necessary in order for the classification to have any value. For example, antecedent conditions to childhood depressions such as parent-child relations should be part of the body of information generated by the classification. Also, predictions about relations with peers, school performance, the likelihood of responding to certain kinds of treatment are some of the variables that should eventuate from a meaningful diagnosis.

Frequently, attribution to children of trait behaviors or labels tends to be an exercise in tautology. We infer the disorder from the symptom and then we say the symptom is produced by the disorder. I think this has been the case in the area of aggressive drive. To temper the exaggerated psychopathologic significance noted by Kanner attached to symptoms observed in a clinical sample, the definition of a disorder such as childhood depression requires experience with an adequate sample representative of a universe of children. This sample should be studied to determine the incidence and distribution of the putatively deviant behavior in the general child population.

To my knowledge, there are no epidemiological studies of depressive symptoms in childhood. There are, however, at least two good epidemiological studies of deviant behavior in children that treat some of the behaviors frequently classified as depressive symptoms. The series of studies done by Lapouse and Monk (1958) and Lapouse (1966) comes to mind. These studies dealt with 482 children, ages 6 to 12, randomly selected from systematically sampled households in Buffalo, New York. Mothers and teachers were interviewed with a closed-end questionnaire. The results showed that over 40% of the children were reported to have seven or more fears or worries, 30% had nightmares, 25% had body manipulations of various kinds, 20% had been enuretic in the recent past, overactivity occurred in approximately 50%, and 10% showed loss of temper one or more times a day. It is noteworthy that these deviant behaviors, which look so alarming in the clinic, occur with fair frequency in the general child population of which this Buffalo sample is probably representative. A statistically significant excess of high scores was found among the 6- to 8-year-old group when compared with the 9- to 12-year-old group, which is important because of the possibility that these behaviors dissipate with time.

The authors conclude, "The strikingly high prevalence of so-called symptomatic behaviors, their excessive presence in younger as contrasted to older children, and the weak association between these behaviors and adjustment give rise to the question whether behavior deviations are truly indicative of psychiatric disorder or whether they occur as transient developmental phe-nomena in essentially normal children."

Increased age was found to be the most important demographic factor associated with the decreased amount of deviation in behavior. Deviant behavior was related to maladjustment but only in the low socioeconomic group. This finding has implications for the definition of childhood depression made on a clinic sample. If that sample is not representative of the distribution of socioeconomic status in the general child population, then the disorder may be social class related.

Another pertinent epidemiological study, reported by Werry and Quay (1971), was concerned with the prevalence of behavior symptoms in younger elementary school children. The purpose of that study was to obtain preval-ence data on 55 behavior symptoms commonly found in child guidance clinic populations as they occur in school children from kindergarten through grade 2. They studied 1,753 children or approximately 96% of the entire population in these three grades in the Urbana, Illinois school system. Again, this rather large sample is probably representative of the general child population, although it did tend toward a middle-class socioeconomic rating. The data were contributed in the form of teachers' ratings on the Quay-Peterson Problem Checklist, an instrument which, comparatively, has been well-researched. Of the 55 symptoms, approximately 16, in my opinion, have been classified by various writers (Cytryn and McKnew, 1972; Hetherington and Martin, 1972; Malmquist, 1975) as symptoms of childhood depression. Now that I have seen Dr. Kovacs' list, I think that all 55 could be used.

For each sex I computed the range and average percentage prevalence of these 16 behaviors associated with depression in this normal population. For the 926 boys in the Werry and Quay (1971) study, the range of prevalence for the 16 behaviors was from 7.2 to 46.3% with a mean of 22%. For the 827 girls I found a range from 4.6 to 41.4% with a mean of 18%. The symptoms for the 16 behaviors are as follows: fixed expression, lack of emotional reactivity; disruptiveness, tendency to annoy others; feelings of inferiority; crying over minor annoyances and hurts; preoccupation, in a world of his own; shyness, bashfulness; lack of self-confidence; fighting; temper tantrums; hypersensitiv-ity, feelings easily hurt; anxiety, chronic general fearfulness; depression, chronic sadness; aloofness; sluggishness, lethargy; nervousness, jitteryness, jumpiness, easily startled; often has physical complaints, headaches, stomachaches.

These data are instructive because they suggest that approximately 20% of the general child population has been reliably judged to possess the symptoms of depressive disorder observed in clinical samples. When compared with the incidence of other childhood disorders, this rate in the general population is quite high. For example, the prevalence of childhood psychosis is estimated in the general population from 0.02 (2/10,000) to 0.008% (8/100,000). In clinical referrals the rate is estimated at 5 to 9%. For mental retardation the estimate in the population is approximately 3%. One of Werry's conclusions is that "the prevalence of many symptoms of psychopathology in the general 5 to 8 year old population is quite high and their individual diagnostic value is therefore very limited."

Inasmuch as these kinds of behaviors tend to become less frequent with age, what we may have, if this 20% rate of depressive symptoms in the child population is at all accurate, is a transient developmental phenomenon that will mostly dissipate if left alone. Even in cases of loss or separation (reduction of available reinforcement), reports (Hetherington and Martin, 1972) indicate that most children recover from what is thought to be a depression-withdrawal phase in several weeks and show normal interest and responsiveness to their environment. Similar results have been found in monkeys who were separated from their mothers (Kaufman and Rosenblum, 1967).

With respect to the methodological considerations Dr. Gittelman discussed in the latter part of her chapter, I would extend the five basic criteria for diagnostic clarity she proposes into a multivariate approach following the Peterson model developed in the early 1960s. The first step would be an adequate sampling of the behaviors of children that would be considered indicators of depression. And this would, I think, start at the clinical level—on the expert level. The second step would be development of a reliable instrument to assess these behaviors in the general population. One technique might be the use of peer nominations. All of the items would be intercorrelated and the resulting matrix factor analyzed. The interrelated clusters would then form factors or underlying dimensions. The factor loading would be obtained for each constituent behavior on the list, which would reveal the extent to which that behavior is related to the underlying dimension. Any unselected child could be placed somewhere on the resulting dimensions depending on the number of depressive behaviors that child manifested. In this model children would not differ qualitatively by type but only quantitatively in terms of the number of behaviors on which they were scored. Thus a child would be placed according to degree of depression on one or more of the factors that eventuated from the factor analysis.

REFERENCES

Cytryn, L., and McKnew, D. H. Proposed classification of childhood depression. *Am. J. Psychiatry*, 129:149–155, 1972.

Hetherington, E. M., and Martin, B. Family interaction and psychopathology in children. In H. C. Quay and J. S. Werry (eds.): *Psychopathological Disorders of Children*. New York, John Wiley & Sons, 1972.

Kanner, L. Do behavioral symptoms always indicate psychopathology? *J. Child Psychol. Psychiatry*, 1:17–25, 1960.

Kaufman, I. C., and Rosenblum, L. A. The reaction to separation in infant monkeys: anaclitic depression and conservation—withdrawal. *Psychosom. Med.*, 29:648–675, 1967.

Lapouse, R. The epidemiology of behavior disorders in children. *Am. J. Dis. Child.*, 111:594–599, 1966.

Lapouse, R., and Monk, M. A. An epidemiologic study of behavior characteristics in children. *Am. J. Public Health,* 48:1134–1144, 1958.

Malmquist, C. P. Depression in childhood. In F. Flach and S. Draghi (eds.): *The Nature and Treatment of Depression.* New York, John Wiley & Sons, 1975.

Quay, H. C. Patterns of aggression, withdrawal and immaturity. In H. C. Quay and J. S. Werry (eds.): *Psychopathological Disorders of Childhood.* New York, John Wiley & Sons, 1972.

Werry, J. S., and Quay, H. C. The prevalence of behavior symptoms in younger elementary school children. *Am. J. Orthopsychiatry,* 41:136–143, 1971.

Depression in Childhood: Diagnosis, Treatment, and Conceptual Models, edited by J. G. Schulterbrandt and A. Raskin. Raven Press, New York, 1977.

Pediatric Psychopharmacology and Childhood Depression

Judith L. Rapoport

Departments of Pediatrics and Psychiatry, Georgetown University School of Medicine, Washington, D.C. 20007

I wish to offer data from the infant field of pediatric psychopharmacology to the new and controversial area of childhood depression as one focus for conceptualizing childhood affective disorder. This chapter is not intended as an argument for pharmacotherapy in childhood. However, some creative uses of drug response have been proposed as a means of syndromal identification (Klein, 1973), and I would like to review some possible similar approaches to childhood depression and suggest avenues for further work.

In particular, the following three areas may sharpen our focus on issues inherent in defining affective illness in early childhood: first, there appears to be a striking difference between the affective response of preadolescent children and that of adults to stimulant drugs and to steroids. Secondly, studies of drug treatment of so-called masked depressions or depressive equivalents may provide a technique for relating an underlying dysphoric mood state to symptom development and/or maintenance. Finally, preliminary clinical reports on pharmacotherapy for "depressed" children may suggest possible clinical subgroupings of these heterogeneous groups as well as designs for future treatment studies.

EFFECTS OF STIMULANT DRUGS AND STEROIDS ON MOOD IN YOUNG CHILDREN

Stimulants have been shown to produce a positive or euphoric mood in approximately 60% of normal adults (Lasagna et al., 1955; Weiss and Laties, 1962); in doses approximating those used on a per kilogram basis with hyperkinetic children, both "activation" and positive mood are reported by normal adults. This euphoric response has been of clinical interest since depressed adults who exhibit a positive mood change with stimulants may be more likely to respond to tricyclic antidepressants (Fawcett et al., 1973), and this euphoric response to amphetamine may be blocked by prior lithium administration (Von Kammen and Murphy, 1975). A body of studies dealing with stimulant drug effects in children is briefly reviewed below.

The child's response to stimulants seems in some contrast to that observed for adults. Eisenberg (1972) has commented on the "remarkable lack of euphoric effect of the stimulants" in children, and that has also been our experience. Some controlled studies have attempted to measure mood and motivational changes; but in behavior-disordered children striking improvement of hyperactive and aggressive behaviors has been seen, although anxiety symptoms may even worsen. Conners and Eisenberg (1963), for example, reporting on stimulant drug treatment of a population of children with behavior disorders, found a nonsignificant trend for listless and apathetic behavior to improve as compared with powerful drug effects on troublesome or demanding behaviors. Anxiety symptoms such as nailbiting and fearfulness worsened, and drug effects on mood *per se* were equivocal; the drug-treated group did report that they felt slightly happier, but this was not striking, and such response may have been produced principally in the older children since the population included children up to age 15.

Conners, Eisenberg, and Barcai (1967) studied motivation in children receiving either amphetamine or placebo. They found a highly significant drug effect on a test battery which seeed to measure a child's "optimism" concerning his performance in a variety of tasks (pencil and paper) and estimates of how well he might do in a variety of physical activities (such as sports). The authors describe this group of response variables as similar to Catell's factor II, or "ego expansiveness," and they feel it may be a useful way of measuring some mood change in middle childhood. However, there does not appear to be a clinical correlate of this effect, and these changes may not have been independent of cognitive changes induced by the drug.

Our attempts (Rapoport et al., 1974) to demonstrate a change in mood, as observed by a structured interview after 6 weeks of stimulant drug or placebo, were completely unsuccessful; responses to a self-concept scale (Piers and Harris, 1963) containing 30 items about self-worth, such as "I do bad things," and "I have a pleasant face," showed no difference at 6 weeks on stimulant or tricyclic drugs compared with placebo. We did obsrve almost universally that grade school children object to considering and/or sharing introspections of this sort. A critical point, therefore, is whether such a negative finding indicates an insensitivity of the rating instrument or reflects a true qualitative difference in affectual response to stimulants. The latter explanation is supported by the fact that children on stimulants often exhibit a striking impression of seriousness or even sadness, even when there is marked clinical benefit from the drugs in other areas of functioning. Sensitive parents and teachers may become concerned about their child's new anhedonic approach to life.

It can (and will) be argued that hyperactive children may differ in their basic capacity to experience pleasure or pain (Wender, 1971) and therefore that this population represents atypical preadolescents. For hyperactive children who continue to use stimulants, mood changes in adolescence have not been formally studied. I have followed a single case of an adolescent girl for whom stimulant drug had to be discontinued at age 16 because of its new effect as a mood elevator, when previously (from ages 8 to 13) the child had exhibited the "typical" noneuphoric response. A similar case has been reported by Mackay et al. (1973) in a paper on the use of stimulants with adolescents with histories of minimal brain dysfunction.

There are no data on the effect of stimulants on mood in normal children because such a study is not ethically feasible. However, Dr. Rachel Gittelman *(personal communication)* examined 29 learning disabled children, otherwise behaviorally normal, who received a mean daily dose of 50 mg methylphenidate, and she found no evidence of mood change on psychiatric interview or teacher rating for this group.

The only other populations of children observed during amphetamine treatment were those described in early uncontrolled studies for whom "stimulation" was noted on amphetamines. Fish (1971) has argued that there is no one optimal type of patient for whom stimulants should be given, and he stresses that stimulation can occur in pediatric populations. These early reports for "neurotic" children given amphetamines are fragmentary and unconvincing that true mood change occurs during stimulant drug treatment.

Bradley and Bowen (1941) reported that of the 19 children who became "stimulated" when given amphetamines, only 12 exhibited an "increased sense of well-being." Interestingly, one child is quoted as saying, "I feel joy in my stomach," suggesting that items of somatic sensation may be useful in mood rating for children. A few children were seen as having increased interest in their surroundings.

The majority of the "stimulated" children, however, fell into two groups: (1) those whose behavior was somewhat bizarre at base line, such as an 8-year-old boy with 2 years of school refusal or a 12-year-old with "fantastic ideas" and long periods of mutism (Bradley and Bowen, 1941; Bender and Cottington, 1942; Bradley, 1950); or (2) children with considerable aggressive symptomatology whose apparent mood change was inferred from decrease in destructive behavior.

It is certainly not clear if any of the hospitalized children described in these early reports would be considered "depressed." Few changes indicating increased involvement and alertness may occur, and measurement of aspiration level, such as that used in the study of Conners and Eisenberg (1963), may be more promising. True euphoric response to stimulants seems extremely rare, however, and this may reflect a real refractoriness of the young child's affective system to these agents.

A second area of interest is the response of preadolescent children to endogenous and exogenous corticosteroids. For adults excessive corticosteroids is highly associated with depression. As many as 75% of adults with Cushing's disease may have depression as a presenting symptom (Williams et al., 1974). Glaser (1953) found that 40% of 222 patients with Cushing's syndrome and 36% of 100 patients treated with corticotropin developed mental changes. One review of psychiatric complications associated with adrenal hyperfunction reported for 94 adults found that over half exhibited severe depression (Fawcett and Bunney, 1967). Primary adrenal hyperplasia is not seen in young children, but 85% of adrenal tumors are found in children under 7 (Mackay, 1975). Furthermore, corticosteroids are in wide use by pediatricians for inflammatory and allergic conditions.

Preliminary data suggest that there is no comparable psychopathological response in children with Cushing's syndrome or in those receiving steroid therapy. One recent textbook specifically notes the rarity of concurrent emotional disturbance in cushingoid children (Eberlain and Winter, 1969). In a series of over 500 cases treated by the Nephrology Unit, Department of Pediatrics, Georgetown Hospital, two cases of psychosis could be recalled. No other behavior changes attributable to drug treatment were noted.

This report might indicate the lack of the psychiatric acumen in the overtaxed pediatric nephrologists; it is apparent, however, that the dramatic and intrusive psychiatric complications of steroid treatment found for adults are not conspicuous with children. The intriguing question then arises whether other nondysphoric behaviors do appear in this group. A survey of the behavioral changes of children undergoing steroid therapy is presently in progress in 23 nephrosis treatment centers treating, collectively, over 2,000 children.

Preliminary impressions (A. Spitzer, *personal communication*) are that although mood changes *per se* are almost unknown, mild insomnia, emotional lability, irritability, or hyperactivity may occur. The question again is whether we are recording the insensitivity of measurers and measuring instruments or true affective stability in this age group. If negative, this preliminary clinical survey would need to be further documented by objective prospective evaluations.

Of course, differential responses to drug between infants and adults might be owing to a variety of factors, such as different absorption and metabolism or excretion of the drug (Mirkin, 1975). Such data are available and should be examined. If mood swings and behavioral changes of clinical significance are found to occur at all, intensive clinical and physiological studies of those children who exhibit drastic and sustained mood alterations would be of interest.

DRUG TREATMENT OF "MASKED DEPRESSION"

A second possible pharmacologic contribution toward defining childhood depression might be in the treatment of the so-called masked depressions.

Among groups of children having enuresis, headache and other somatic complaints, school failure, hyperactivity, and antisocial behavior, there is commonly assumed to exist a subgroup of children who are primarily depressed. This is a critical question since most would agree that striking persistent dysphoria is rare in early childhood, whereas these other difficulties are extremely common and, indeed, account for most of the symptoms seen in child guidance clinic populations. There have been a few reports in which antidepressant medication has been used with these groups.

If antidepressants can be shown to alter mood in children, this may provide an important strategy for relating mood change and symptom production or maintenance.

Enuresis

Enuresis is a common condition of childhood for which no certain incidence is available because definitions of the problem (duration and frequency) vary from study to study. One recent whole population study (Rutter et al., 1970), however, reported an overall incidence of 5% for 10- and 11-year-olds on the Isle of Wight. Although enuresis occurs as an isolated symptom (Lapouse and Monk, 1958), the Isle of Wight study found a strong association between enuresis and other behavior problems: 9% of "high score" children and 1% of "low score" children had enuresis as a problem. However, enuretic children were not likely to have any specific type of associated disorder—antisocial, neurotic, and developmental problems were all common for the enuretic group. Enuretic children, as a group, have also been found to have disturbance in arousal patterns during sleep (Broughton, 1968), indicating a general disturbance in CNS function.

The responses of approximately 70% of enuretic children to tricyclic antidepressants (Poussaint and Ditman, 1967) have been of considerable practical and theoretical interest. Although the tricyclics are known to exert multiple effects (anticholinergic, effect on bladder, and alteration in arousal patterns during sleep), the question has been raised about the relation of an effect on mood to the effect on enuresis. Poussaint and Ditman did not examine behavior disturbances for their group.

A more recent double-blind study (Werry et al., 1976) of imipramine treatment of 24 enuretic boys included behavioral evaluation: 18 of the boys were considered normal, 6 were seen as mildly disturbed. There was no evidence that the latter group responded more favorably than the former to antidepressants. There were reports of "happier, more cooperative" behavior for the drug versus the placebo group, but this had no relation to the antienuretic effect. Werry and co-workers' sample obtained an improvement rate (60%) with antidepressant drug similar to that found by Poussaint and Ditman, despite the lack of associated problems.

One study, unfortunately including only a small number of children, comparing problem and nonproblem enuretics given imipramine suggested that imipramine was more effective for children with less history of associated neurotic behavior. Ritvo et al. (1969) found that seven enuretic boys, ages 8 to 10, could be differentiated by arousal pattern of enuresis (neurotic) and nonarousal pattern (nonneurotic). This latter nonarousal, nonneurotic group had the better response to imipramine.

It would be of considerable interest to extend Ritvo's study comparing larger numbers of neurotic and nonneurotic enuretic children. If, as Ritvo indicates, neurotic children respond poorly to imipramine, a controlled trial of another drug such as a monoamine oxidase (MAO) inhibitor might be justified. It would be important to see what happened to the enuretic symptoms once mood alterations were effected by drug treatment.

There has not yet been a satisfactory controlled study demonstrating the beneficial effect of MAO inhibitors on mood in young children, as discussed below. Nevertheless, it is most interesting that Frommer (1968) has indicated in an uncontrolled clinical report that when mood is altered favorably by MAO inhibitors given for "enuretic depressives," the enuresis usually does not change. The preponderance of boys in this group and the continuation of enuresis even after favorable treatment of the depression raise the possibility that one subgroup of so-called masked depressions of childhood includes physiologically immature children with both emotional lability and enuresis as manifestations of a common underlying difficulty. Frommer has suggested such a distinction.

Hyperactivity

Hyperactive children, as a group, have not been found to have a high incidence of relatives with affective disorder (Cantwell, 1972; Stewart and Morrison, 1973), unlike that where genetic associations with alcoholism and hysteria have been described. However, the existence of some subgroup of depressed hyperactive children is generally assumed (Cytryn and McKnew, 1972), and several follow-up studies have stressed the low self-esteem and depressive affect for this group in adolescence.

Because of this notion, we were interested in whether a group of hyperactive children responding to tricyclic antidepressants would be characterized by, for example, a family history of depressive illness or by coexisting anxiety. Our data provided no support for this. First, the tricyclics were not very effective.

Secondly, in spite of our impression that the (very few) good responders were more anxious than the tricyclic nonresponders, another double-blind study did not confirm this. In their series, Waizer et al. (1974) found aggressive hyperactive children to be the best responders. Response to tricyclics was not predicted by family history of depression or by ratings of current situational stress. Thus, in the heterogeneous population of hyperactive children, we could reach no conclusion about a drug-responsive symptom cluster or a responsive subgroup.

It is of anecdotal interest that of the 6 children (out of 76 in the sample) still on imipramine at 2-year follow-up, 4 had had family separations by divorce, whereas this was noted for only 8 of the other 70 children ($\chi^2 = 12$, $p < 0.001$). This is a unique illustration of drug response predicting a follow-up event. Whether or not the children were maintained on antidepressants because the pediatrician assumed that such familial stress was imminent can not be determined.

An alternate and reasonable interpretation of the coexistence of dysphoric ideation and other symptomatology is that the dysphoria represents a demoralized response to a primary handicapping condition. In a 2-year follow-up study (Riddle and Rapoport, 1976) of hyperactive children, our aim was to examine the relation between symptom control during the 2-year period and depressive ideation at follow-up. We expected that for our hyperactive population, depressive mood would appear secondary to the continued negative interpersonal interaction and/or academic failure these children encounter. We used the Cytryn and McKnew (1972) definition of depression—for which statements of overt expression of helplessness and worthlessness were recorded, scored, and evaluated—as well as projective stories given to 4 Thematic Apperception Test cards. An interrater reliability of 0.94 was obtained between two clinical psychologists for ratings of depressive content of stories given by patients and controls. The hyperactive group was strikingly more depressed than the age- and sex-matched control population. No significant correlation was obtained within the patient group between ratings of depression at base line and at 2-year follow-up. A weak correlation ($r = 0.34$; $p < 0.01$) was obtained with age and ratings of depression for the follow-up sample: older children were seen as more depressed. However, our expectations that depressive symptomatology would be predicted by background factors, onset and duration of hyperactivity, family stress, academic failure, or poor control of hyperactivity symptoms by medication was not confirmed. Children maintained in good control on stimulant drug (86% of an initial randomly assigned group of good responders) were rated as depressed as the children who had stopped taking the drug or who had been maintained inconsistently in poor control.

In summary, the findings were equivocal; there was considerably more depressive ideation in the hyperactive sample, but we did not establish that this was secondary to other concurrent problems. It is possible that emotional lability with depressed or helpless fantasy may be a feature of the common underlying condition labeled "minimal brain dysfunction." Other follow-up studies of treatment of "depressive equivalents" might profitably examine the relation between symptom control or amelioration and mood with, hopefully, clearer results.

Headache

There is clinical consensus that depressed children may present with multiple somatic complaints, including stomachaches and headaches. In a study of children suffering from headache, Ling et al. (1970) used relatively specific criteria for depression: mood change, social withdrawal, poor school performance, recent aggressive behavior, self-deprecation, lack of energy, school phobia, weight loss, and anorexia. Of 25 children undergoing diagnostic evaluation for chronic headache, 10 met these criteria for depression and 9 were treated with tricyclic antidepressants (doses unspecified). The change in frequency of headaches, presumably a criterion for improvement, is not given; Ling et al. report that the 9 from the depressed group who were treated with antidepressants all did well and state that "symptoms disappeared." If controlled studies demonstrate positive mood alteration with tricyclics for children, then a controlled study of drug treatment of depressed children presenting with chronic headache would be worthwhile.

Anxiety

The relation between anxiety and depression is not clear with respect to adult depression: there is evidence for a separate group of patients for whom anxiety symptoms predominate (Roth et al., 1972). However, in the much noted absence of overt depressive symptomatology in children, both phobias and chronic anxiety are important subgroups in clinical descriptions of childhood depression. Anxious or phobic groups are also likely to have a preponderance of girls, resembling the distribution of adult depressive illness.

The only controlled study of drug treatment of anxiety in childhood is that by Gittelman-Klein and Klein (1971) of imipramine treatment of school phobia. In that placebo-controlled, double-blind study, 35 school-phobic children, ages 6 to 14, were followed for 6 weeks and given either imipramine or placebo concurrent with supportive nondrug therapy. Imipramine was superior in inducing school return and in global therapeutic efficacy. The specific item of "observed depression" was also significantly improved with drug compared with placebo. Self-ratings of improvement by the child were most successful in differentiating between drug and placebo treatment groups, although this had no simple relation to school return. The authors do not interpret these results as indicating school phobia to have a primary "depressive" basis. They based their reasoning on the absence of anhedonia in their population, as well as on the demonstration of other drug-responsive anxiety states in adults without overt depression (Klein, 1964). Finally, there is no clear follow-up relationship between childhood phobia and depressive disorder in later life.

Although the school phobic's response to tricyclic antidepressants may not indicate underlying depression, it is of interest that there was a positive mood change with drug, even if this change had no significant relationship to symptom change.

A more common anxiety seen in middle childhood, that of overconcern about external judgment (peer acceptance or school grades), might seem a more fruitful clinical variable to investigate as a precursor of adult depression. For those stressing a superego formulation of depressions in middle childhood, this group of symptoms might be expected to respond to antidepressants, and such a study is waiting to be undertaken.

In addition to clinical pharmacologic studies, animal studies might be useful for investigating affective change and early symptom development. If prior treatment with antidepressants in infant monkeys blocked the initial sequence of protest and despair, then the development of later fearful or isolate behavior could also be followed. Such a study might provide a means for separating the cognitive from affective components in the development of infant grief and mourning states or later "phobic" or overanxious behavior.

DRUG TREATMENT OF "DEPRESSION"

The largest number of reports of antidepressant drug treatment deal with heterogeneous groups of patients described in for the most part uncontrolled trials and not employing objective criteria for improvement. Weinberg et al. (1973) diagnosed depression in a group of 42 children selected from a total population of 72 seen in an educational diagnostic center. Diagnostic criteria included decline in school work, dysphoric mood, and overt statements indicating low self-esteem. Drug treatment was recommended for 35, of whom 19 received treatment. Marked or moderate improvement was described for 18 of the 19, whereas a contrast group of untreated depressed children were described as unchanged. This is one of the more careful and convincing studies.

Frommer (1967, 1968, 1972) has reported the largest series of "depressed" children treated with psychoactive drugs. Her various depressive subgroups have all been treated with antidepressants, and some preliminary impressions of treatment response emerge from her reports. The subgroup of 54 enuretic depressives (31 boys and 23 girls) (1968) had a relatively lower rate of good response [41% compared with over 70% for "mood" depressives ($N = 74$) and phobic depressives ($N = 62$, 22 boys and 40 girls)]. The persistence of enuresis has been discussed previously.

These less-satisfactory treatment results are similar to that of 31% found for 74 children termed "neurotics" who do not have depressed affect. This latter group characterized by speech disorder, congenital abnormalities, and somatic complaints is difficult to relate to our usual categories, but given the high placebo response of outpatient child guidance clinic populations (Eisenberg et al., 1961), the low response rate of these groups would best be labeled as "nonresponse" for the purpose of this survey.

In her double-blind crossover study of 32 cases divided approximately equally between "mood" and "phobic" depressives, Frommer (1967) compared phenelzine and chlordiazepoxide with phenobarbital and placebo. She interpreted the results as showing the superiority of MAO inhibitors and tranquilizers over sedatives and reported equally good response in both the phobic and depressed group. There are several methodologic problems with the study because treatment received first was most effective, and phenobarbital may have had adverse effects on mood. Frommer (1972) also distinguishes between aggressive and nonaggressive preschool depressed children; she reports that the aggressive group is more likely to require concomitant treatment. As with the enuretic group, the aggressive group is predominantly male.

Kuhn and Kuhn (1972), describing antidepressant treatment for a series of 100 preadolescent children, comment that good responders are likely to have a "mature EEG" as well as a positive family history of affective disorder. The dosage of drug and criteria for diagnosis are not given, but some symptoms for inclusion (morning tiredness) are stated.

Other writers (Polvan and Cebiroglu, 1972; Lelord et al., 1972) present less-specific clinical descriptive data and also endorse antidepressant treatment. The consensus among them is that both tricyclic antidepressants and MAO inhibitors are effective agents for a variety of young children, particularly for those exhibiting dysphoric or phobic symptoms.

The idea that congenitally deviant, immature children or those with learning or speech disturbance may be nonresponsive is important, and this distinction would create an important contrast group in a double-blind study. Lucas et al. (1965) carried out a double-blind crossover study of amitriptyline with 14 hospitalized children aged 10 to 15. Only 4 of this group were diagnosed as neurotic; the rest were labeled as schizophrenic or as having a personality disorder. A significant difference was obtained between drug and placebo for ratings of both global improvement and response to controls; the lack of specificity of drug response is most striking in this study.

It is evident from the above that no clear positive antidepressant drug effect or symptom specific for children selected for dysphoria has been demonstrated. In view of a probable placebo response of 60% for outpatient neurotic children (Eisenberg et al., 1961), a controlled drug trial would need relatively large populations in order to establish a significant drug effect; such a study would be worthwhile, especially in view of an apparent ongoing use of antidepressants with children.

Lithium Treatment in Children

Annell (1969*a,b*) has presented extensive use of lithium in children and adolescents who manifested a variety of symptoms, including flagrant psychosis, but having in common a periodic course. In one series, 11 of 12 children responded with marked clinical change. Gram and Rafaelson (1972), in a double-blind, controlled study of 18 inpatients with the diagnosis of psychosis since at least age 5, found that many symptoms responded to lithium, compared with placebo, but the results were by no means dramatic.

Two controlled studies have not found lithium useful for hyperactive children (Whitehead and Clark, 1970; Greenhill et al., 1973), although possible responses for individual cases were suggested. In a search for a lithium-responsive subgroup, Dyson and Barcai (1970) reported two cases of hyperactive children who had a lithium-responding parent. Their clinical data are not convincing: one child required concomitant continued use of stimulants, and no control periods were observed. However, the idea of a drug-responsive subgroup selected on the basis of positive parental treatment response may be a useful model for future studies and may prove more rewarding than subgrouping by symptom cluster. It must be stressed, however, that as lithium may be effective in a variety of disorders, positive response should not be equated with a diagnosis of manic-depressive disease in childhood (Schou, 1972).

SUMMARY

In summary, a survey of these early reports on antidepressant drug use in childhood suggests future work but provides no conclusions about drug efficacy or about the validity of a concept of childhood depression. As one argument for pursuing such drug studies may be that antidepressants are already in general use with children, the current usage of antidepressant drugs by pediatricians and child psychiatrists in the United States should be surveyed. If use is indeed widespread, then clinical guidelines are badly needed. Possible predictors of drug response should include family history of affective illness and drug response, as has recently been stressed elsewhere (Ommen and Motulsky, 1972; Pardue, 1975). Descriptive reports suggest that a cluster of symptoms of hyperactivity, aggressivity, speech disturbance, enuresis, "congenital abnormalities," and abnormal EEG might predict a nonresponsive "minimal brain dysfunction" group.

Studies should also be made of the behavioral response of children to such drugs as steroids, which are known to produce affective disturbance in adults. In the area of experimental depression research, the primate infant's affective response to separation might be pharmacologically manipulated with antidepressants as part of development studies of later behavioral deviance. If controlled studies establish the efficacy of antidepressant drugs in dysphoric children, then the demonstration of a significant relation between mood alteration and changes in manifestation of "depressive equivalents" would be clinically convincing. Such clinically based pharmacologic studies will support further conceptual efforts concerning depression in early childhood.

REFERENCES

Annell, A. L. Lithium in the treatment of children and adolescents. *Acta Psychiatr. Scand. Suppl.*, 207:19–30, 1969*a*.

Annell, A. L. Manic-depressive illness in children and effect of treatment with lithium carbonate. *Acta Paedopsychiatr. (Basel)*, 36:292–301, 1969*b*.

Bender, L., and Cottington, F. The use of amphetamine sulfate (benzedrine) in child psychiatry. *Am. J. Psychiatry*, 99:116–121, 1942.

Bradley, C. Benzedrine and dexedrine in the treatment of children's behavior disorders. *Pediatrics*, 5:24–36, 1950.

Bradley, C., and Bowen, M. Amphetamine (benzedrine) therapy of children's behavior disorders. *Am. J. Orthopsychiatry*, 11:92–103, 1941.

Broughton, R. J. Sleep disorders: Disorders of arousal? *Science*, 159:1070–1077, 1968.

Cantwell, D. P. Psychiatric illness in the families of hyperactive children. *Arch. Gen. Psychiatry*, 27:414–417, 1972.

Conners, C. K., and Eisenberg, L. The effects of methylphenidate on symptomatology and learning in disturbed children. *Am. J. Psychiatry*, 120:459–466, 1963.

Conners, C. K., Eisenberg, L., and Barcai, A. Effect of dextroamphetamine on children. *Arch. Gen. Psychiatry*, 17:478–485, 1967.

Cytryn, L., and McKnew, D. H. Proposed classification of childhood depression. *Am. J. Psychiatry*, 129:63–69, 1972.

Dyson, W. L., and Barcai, A. Treatment of children of lithium responding parents. *Curr. Ther. Res.*, 12:286–290, 1970.

Eberlain, W. R., and Winter, J. S. Cushing's syndrome in childhood. In L. I. Gardner (ed.): *Endocrine and Genetic Diseases of Childhood*. New York, Harper & Row, pp. 428–436, 1969.

Eisenberg, G. L., Cytryn, L., and Molling, P. The effectiveness of psychotherapy alone and in conjunction with perphenazine or placebo in the treatment of neurotic and hyperkinetic children. *Am. J. Psychiatry*, 117:1088–1093, 1961.

Eisenberg, L. The clinical use of stimulant drugs in children. *Pediatrics*, 49:709–715, 1972.

Fawcett, J., Mass, J., and Dekirmenjian, H. Depression and MHPG excretion: Response to dextroamphetamine and tricyclic antidepressants. *Arch. Gen. Psychiatry*, 26:246–251, 1973.

Fawcett, J. A., and Bunney, W. E. Pituitary adrenal function and depression. *Arch. Gen. Psychiatry*, 16:517–535, 1967.

Fish, B. The "one child, one drug" myth of stimulants in hyperkinesis. *Arch. Gen. Psychiatry*, 25:193–203, 1971.

Frommer, E. A. Treatment of childhood depression with antidepressant drugs. *Br. Med. J.*, 1:729–732, 1967.

Frommer, E. A. Depressive illness in childhood. *Br. J. Psychiatry*, Special Pub. #2:117–136, 1968.

Frommer, E. A. Indications for antidepressant treatment with special reference to depressed preschool children. In A. L. Annell (ed.): *Depressive States in Childhood and Adolescence*. New York, John Wiley & Sons, pp. 449–454, 1972.

Gittelman-Klein, R., and Klein, D. F. Controlled imipramine treatment of school phobia. *Arch. Gen. Psychiatry*, 25:204–207, 1971.

Glaser, G. H. The pituitary gland in relation to cerebral metabolism and metabolic disorders of the nervous system. *Res. Publ. Assoc. Res. Nerv. Ment. Dis.*, 32:21–39, 1953.

Gram, L. F., and Rafaelsen, O. J.: Lithium treatment of psychotic children and adolescents. *Acta Psychiatr. Scand.*, 48:253–260, 1972.

Greenhill, L. L., Rieder, R. O., Wender, P. H., et al. Lithium carbonate in the treatment of hyperactive children. *Arch. Gen. Psychiatry*, 28:636–640, 1973.

Klein, D. Delineation of two drug-responsive anxiety syndromes. *Psychopharmacologia*, 5:397–408, 1964.

Klein, D. F. Drug therapy as a means of syndromal identification and nosological revision. In J. O. Cole (ed.): *Psychopathology and Psychopharmacology.* Baltimore, Johns Hopkins University Press, pp. 143–160, 1973.

Kuhn, V., and Kuhn, R. Drug therapy for depression in children. In A. L. Annell (ed.): *Depressive States in Childhood and Adolescence.* New York, John Wiley & Sons, pp. 455–459, 1972.

Lapouse, R., and Monk, M. A. An epidemiologic study of the behaviour characteristics in children. *Am. J. Public Health,* 48:1134–1144, 1958.

Lasagna, L., Van Felsinger, J. M., and Beecher, H. K. Drug induced mood changes in man: (1) Observations on healthy subjects, chronically ill patients and postaddicts. *J.A.M.A.,* 157:1006–1020, 1955.

Lelord, G., Etienne, T., and Veauvy, N. Action de l'opipramol (G 33.040) dans les symptomes depressifs de l'enfance et de l'adolescence. In A. L. Annell (ed.): *Depressive States in Childhood and Adolescence.* New York, John Wiley & Sons, pp. 473–478, 1972.

Ling, W., Oftedal, G., and Weinberg, W. Depressive illness in childhood presenting as severe headache. *Am. J. Dis. Child.,* 120:122–124, 1970.

Lucas, A. R., Lockett, H. J., and Grimm, F. Amitriptyline in childhood depressions. *Dis. Nerv. Syst.,* 26:105–110, 1965.

Mackay, M. C., Beck, L., and Taylor, R. Methylphenidate for adolescents with minimal brain dysfunction. *N.Y. State J. Med.,* 73:550–554, 1973.

Mackay, V. (ed.): *Nelson Textbook of Pediatrics,* Ed. 10. Philadelphia, W. B. Saunders Co., pp. 1326–1346, 1975.

Mirkin, B. L. Placental transfer, fetal localization, and neonatal disposition of drugs. *Anesthesiology,* 43:156–170, 1975.

Ommen, G. S., and Motulsky, A. G. Psycho-pharmacogenetics. In A. R. Kaplan (ed.): *Genetic Factors in "Schizophrenia."* Springfield, Ill., Charles C Thomas, 1972.

Pardue, L. Familial unipolar depressive illness: A pedigree study. *Am. J. Psychiatry,* 132:970–972, 1975.

Piers, E. V., and Harris, D. B. Age and other correlates of self-concept in children. *J. Educ. Psychol.,* 55:91–95, 1963.

Polvan, O., and Cebiroglu, R. Treatment with psychopharmacologic agents in childhood depressions. In A. L. Annell (ed.): *Depressive States in Childhood and Adolescence.* New York, John Wiley & Sons, pp. 467–472, 1972.

Poussaint, A. F., and Ditman, K. S. A controlled study of imipramine (Tofranil) in the treatment of childhood enuresis. *J. Pediatr.,* 67:283–290, 1967.

Rapoport, J. L., Quinn, P. O., Bradbard, G., et al. Imipramine and methylphenidate treatments of hyperactive boys. *Arch. Gen. Psychiatry,* 30:789–793, 1974.

Riddle, D., and Rapoport, J. L. A two year follow-up of 78 hyperactive boys: Classroom behavior and peer acceptance. *J. Nerv. Ment. Dis.,* 162:126–134, 1976.

Ritvo, E. R., Ornitz, E. M., Gotlieb, F., et al. Arousal and non arousal enuretic events. *Am. J. Psychiatry,* 126:77–84, 1969.

Roth, P., Gurney, C., Garside, R., et al. Studies in the classification of affective disorders: The relationship between anxiety states and depressive illnesses. *Br. J. Psychiatry,* 121:147–166, 1972.

Rutter, M., Tizard, J., and Whitmore, K. (ed.): *Education, Health and Behavior.* New York, John Wiley & Sons, 1970.

Schou, M. Lithium in psychiatric therapy and prophylaxis. A review with special regard to its use in children. In A. L. Annell (ed.): *Depressive States in Childhood and Adolescence.* New York, John Wiley & Sons, pp. 479–487, 1972.

Stewart, M. A., and Morrison, J. R. Affective disorder among the relatives of hyperactive children. *J. Child Psychol. Psychiatry,* 14:209–212, 1973.

Von Kammen, D., and Murphy, D. L. Attenuation of the euphoriant and activating effects of d- and l-amphetamine by lithium carbonate treatment. *Psychopharmacologia,* 44:215–224, 1975.

Waizer, J., Hoffman, S. P., Polizos, P., et al. Outpatient treatment of hyperactive school children with imipramine. *Am. J. Psychiatry,* 131:587–591, 1974.

Weinberg, W., Rutman, J., Sullivan, L., et al. Depression in children referred to an educational diagnostic center: Diagnosis and treatment. *J. Pediatr.,* 83:1065–1072, 1973.

Weiss, B., and Laties, V. G. Enhancement of human performance by caffeine and the amphetamines. *Pharmacol. Rev.*, 14:1–36, 1962.

Wender, P. *Minimal Brain Dysfunction in Children*. New York, Wiley-Interscience, 1971.

Werry, J. S., Dowrick, P., and Lampen, E. L. Imipramine in enuresis—psychological and physiological effects. *J. Child Psychol. Psychiatry (in press)*.

Whitehead, P. L., and Clark, L. D. Effect of lithium carbonate, placebo and thioridazine on hyperactive children. *Am. J. Psychiatry,* 127:824–825, 1970.

Williams, G. H., Dluhy, R. G., and Thorn, G. W. Diseases of the adrenal cortex. In M. W. Wintrobe, *Harrison's Principles of Internal Medicine, Ed. 7*. M. W. Wintrobe, G. W. Thorn, and R. D. Adams (eds.): New York, McGraw Hill, pp. 499–505, 1974.

Discussion of Dr. Rapoport's Chapter:
Pediatric Psychopharmacology and Childhood Depression

C. Keith Conners

Western Psychiatric Institute and Clinics, University of Pittsburgh School of Medicine, Pittsburgh, Pennsylvania 15261

The first thing I would like to comment on is the stimulants in hyperactive children. I learned recently from reading one of Dr. Anthony's many new books that when Charles Bradley was first exploring the use of amphetamine (Benzedrine®) in children, his first idea about the action of the stimulants was simply that the children had a dysphoric mood, and that most of the behavior problems stemmed from dysphoria either as an accompaniment to their basic problem or as a cause of their bad behavior. The effect of amphetamine in alleviating a large percentage of their behavior symptoms was that it improved the mood by "increasing their sense of well-being," as he put it. They were able to cope with school and to give up many of the symptoms that he thought were in effect attempts to cope. In other words, this is an early masked depression hypothesis.

Bradley gave up that idea because there was no consistent evidence that mood did in fact improve, and he substituted a notion that instead the drug somehow increased tonic inflow to the cortex and therefore created a greater degree of cortical inhibition.

In our studies we have found few overt changes in mood in these children. That is, they do not report that they feel high. Parents in general don't say they look high. On the contrary, mood comments tend to be that the children appear a little sadder. Many of the children have the amphetamine look, the masked facies, the peripheral autonomic effect that misleads people into thinking they are sad. They look as though they have a bad hangover. This doesn't mean that they actually feel sad, but perhaps 10 to 15% of such children respond in a most dramatic way. Ounsted (1955) noticed this even in a series of epileptic children treated with stimulants who appeared to have instant superego and resembled adults with clinical depressions.

Children who respond dramatically are weepy, sad, and listless, and they express feelings of mournfulness and hopelessness. They become quite retarded in their motor activity, and this is usually why parents dislike the treatment. We have uniformly taken such children off medication because the side effects are worse than the original problem. I have never found anything that predicts that response. We looked for a history of family illnesses of various kinds including depression, and that was not consistent either, but it is a phenomenon that needs investigation because these children do not simply become sedated or overmedicated. This is not like the overmedication response in a child who responds at a lower dose. It is some kind of physiological reversal, and that is a good model of depressive illness. The sort of criteria one can use is such that where a reprimand previously had no effect, even slight criticism provokes such a child to tears and feelings of guilt. Several children in effect said almost overnight, "I don't know why everybody picks on me. I don't know why I'm so bad. I know I do lots of bad things," etc. In other words, they verbalized depressing thoughts that they had never verbalized before.

We usually exclude this group from the series because they are inappropriate. Perhaps we misdiagnose them in some obscure way, but it's an interesting biochemical response that may be caused by sudden depletion of catecholamines or some related effect.

No one has systematically examined the issue of sleep disturbance in children treated with amphetamines, but there are a number of interesting allusions. Mendelwicz and Klotz (1974) point out that enuretics frequently have sleep disturbances. In Frommer's (1967, 1968) series she describes early morning waking in one of her subgroups, and she takes this as an indication for the use of amitriptyline (Elavil®). There may be a group of children who have a disturbance of autonomic regulation and central arousal that produces in addition to their behavioral symptoms disturbances of sleep and disturbances of mood.

But again, taking adult depression as a hypothesis about how to look at the phenomenon in children, one might ask, "Are there children who from quite early in life have disturbances in their sleep pattern or in their vegetative cycles generally?"

One is struck with the number of children who come not only with fitful sleep, restlessness in sleep, and disturbances of appetite, but also with other signs suggesting that the whole autonomic system is poorly regulated. I think this may be an area in which to look in terms of drug response.

The studies on lithium unfortunately are poorly done. We can dismiss, I think, for the reason Dr. Rapoport stated, the Dyson and Barcai (1970) study. The most interesting cases are in the series recorded by Annel (1969, 1972) in Sweden. Eight or ten of these case reports are quite intriguing. The children were from mixed diagnostic categories—one appeared catatonic, another seemed to be retarded. Some were schizophrenic children, most of whom had not shown in their younger years any depressive picture. Yet when they reached adolescence they were treated with lithium on the grounds that their parents had a history of bipolar affective illness. Annell reports dramatic changes in that uncontrolled series. Although the study was uncontrolled, it has some weight because the symptoms were severe in institutionalized children who suddenly became normal, as it were. One can't help thinking that perhaps in those children gross psychopathology was really a learned or secondary reaction to some more primary disturbances, which when treated allowed the secondary symptoms to disappear. The possibility of doing a genetic study intrigues me.

The study of Weinberg et al. (1973) is probably the best study in the literature on antidepressants, and the study is not exactly uncontrolled. The authors did not have a randomly selected control group, but they had 19 kids who I believe elected to go on drug therapy, and another group who either refused or for some other reason could not go on drug therapy, and the improvement rate was 18 out of 19 in the treated group and approximately 3 out of 20 in the other group. In other words, the control was not blind, but it sounds very convincing the way it is described.

The other thing that makes the study of Weinberg et al. unique is that like Dr. Cytryn's study, the investigation included children who were carefully selected on the basis of clearly defined depressive criteria, and again, not just depressive mood but the whole course of the illness seemed to suggest that the children reflected a different entity.

One other thing that really relates to something that Dr. Malmquist touched on is the role of loss in depressive illness and how it relates to drug treatment. We examined our data on hyperactive kids in terms of whether there was a differential response if the child had been a foster child, had a lost parent, or showed some other clear antecedent, and we found no differences. However, Perris (1976) summarized a number of studies and found that 16 or 17% of adult depressives had a history of parental loss. Such a small number indicates that loss itself does not lead to uniform depression.

Why do some people who have loss become classic depressives? The answer I would suggest is biological because if you divide patients into those with and without a family history, the rate goes up rather dramatically. A study by Felix Brown (1972) at the Hampstead Clinic in England reports approximately 43% loss of either parent, but that is the only study of its kind. Most other studies report rather small frequency overall for adult depressives who have had a significant loss. The incidence of loss in a group of depressed children may be significant, but it represents only a small proportion of the total number of kids.

Thus, loss is a variable that seems to lead to depression in some people, and I suggest that it must interact with some other variable. Something else in addition to loss must be present in order to lead to persistent and severe depression. Every child experiences depressive affects in mourning after a loss, but only some children continue to experience such affects for a pro-longed period, and only some of those in later life have a depressive breakdown.

The psychopharmacology of depression is in very early stages. Frommer's (1967, 1968) work is totally confusing to me. She is the only person who has a large series of what she calls depressive children. She divides them into three categories and claims that they differ in response to MAO inhibitors, tricyclic antidepressants, and minor tranquilizers. But looking in detail at her paper, it's impossible to tell whether those three groups really differ in a systematic way and how they are selected.

I suggest that after developing firm criteria and selecting a group of depressed children with different antecedent backgrounds and different genetic histories, one should then divide those groups into drug and nondrug treatment categories to see if there is a differential response. I doubt that studying an unselected group for response to drug treatment is going to tell much because, as Rachel Gittelman pointed out, the drugs have multiple actions—that a child's condition improves with a certain drug doesn't mean that he has any kind of biological deficit specific to that drug. Lithium, for example, is not simply a prophylactic antidepressant, but it has some sedative effects. Also, amitriptyline and all of the tricyclics have more than one action so that one cannot conclude that the effect is specifically antidepressant in any simple way.

Except for the remarkable finding of kids who become clinically depressed with stimulants, there isn't much to be said about the role of psychopharmacology at this point, but if one were going to do studies on this he would need to delineate subgroups very carefully before trying different medications.

REFERENCES

Annell, A.-L. Manic depressive illness in children and effect of treatment with lithium carbonate. *Acta Paedopsychiatr.*, 36:292–301, 1969.

Annell, A.-L. (ed.): *Depressive States in Childhood and Adolescence*. Stockholm, Almquist & Wiksell, 1972.

Brown, F. Depression and childhood bereavement. In: A.-L. (ed.): *Depressive States in Childhood and Adolescence*. Stockholm, Almquist & Wiksell, pp. 35–44, 1972.

Dyson, W. L., and Barcai, A. Treatment of children of lithium-responding parents. *Curr. Ther. Res.*, 12:286–290, 1970.

Frommer, E. Treatment of childhood depression with antidepressant drugs. *Br. Med. J.*, 5542:729–732, 1967.

Frommer, E. Depressive illness in childhood. *Br. J. Psychiatry*, 2:117–136, 1968.

Mendelwicz, J., and Klotz, J. Primary enuresis and affective illness (a letter). *Lancet*, 1(7860):733, 1974.

Ounsted, C. The hyperkinetic syndrome in epileptic children. *Lancet*, 269(2):303–311, 1955.

Perris, C. Frequency and hereditary aspects of depression. In D. M. Gallant and G. M. Simpson (eds.): *Depression: Behavioral, Biochemical, Diagnostic and Treatment Concepts*. Holliswood, N.Y., Spectrum Press, pp. 75–95, 1976.

Weinberg, W., Rutman, J., Sullivan, L., Penick, E., et al. Depression in children referred to an educational diagnostic center. Diagnosis and treatment—preliminary report. *J. Pediatr.*, 83:1065–1072, 1973.

Conceptual Models

Depression in Childhood: Diagnosis, Treatment, and Conceptual Models, edited by J. G. Schulterbrandt and A. Raskin. Raven Press, New York, 1977.

Animal Behavioral/Biological Models Relevant to Depressive and Affective Disorders in Humans

William T. McKinney, Jr.

Department of Psychiatry, University of Wisconsin Medical School, Madison, Wisconsin 53706

INTRODUCTION

Most early studies in animal psychopathology suffered from an inability to demonstrate relevance beyond the highly specific situation in which they were produced and from a premature application of human clinical labels. Consequently, several writers expressed great skepticism concerning the relevance of animal behavioral models of psychopathology to human disorders. Kubie (1939) was a leading spokesman for those psychiatrists who refused to accept animal models. He states, "The imitation in animals of the emotional states which attain neurosis in man is not the experimental production of the essence of neuroses itself." For Kubie, behavior that is observable is only to be interpreted as "the sign language" of an underlying symbolic disorder which is the real core of psychopathology. He stressed that animals do not have symbolic capacity, and therefore it is impossible to produce a true neurotic or psychotic state in nonhumans. This criticism, if true, would preclude the use of any nonhuman subjects for the study of human psychopathology. However, the assumption that higher-order primates do not have symbolic capacity is being seriously questioned (Premack, 1970) as, of course, is the belief that overt behavior is only a symptom of an underlying symbolic disorder which is the real core of psychopathology. The early literature in the area of animal modeling is difficult to read, and there was poor communication between the experimental workers and the clinicians with regards to its relevance and comparability. There were severe methodological problems and little preciseness in the use of labels.

Given these difficulties, it is even more amazing how rapidly the field has progressed since 1966 when Senay put forward the concept of an animal model that would reflect human depression. He used puppies and separation from the experimenter was a precipitating event, and Senay described depressive symptomatology that lasted for 2 months until the puppies were reunited with the investigator.

Seligman and Maier (1967) then presented an analysis of the response of dogs to electric shock. They worked on two premises of learning and the relationships that produced learning, acquisition and extinction. A third relationship was proposed, that of independence between events. The term they used was "learned helplessness" defined as the perception (or learning) of independence between the animals' responses and the aversive event whether it was withdrawal or presentation. More specifically, if the dogs had had an initial experience in a situation where they had no control over reinforcers, they subsequently failed to attempt control in the same situation later, even though their behavior could have then controlled the reinforcers. Later papers by this group reported that the pathological behavior that resulted from inescapable trauma was alleviated by having the animals repeatedly respond to the event which terminated the shock (Seligman, 1973). They speculated that, like dogs, humans also become passive in situations where they cannot, or feel that they cannot, mitigate or control future traumatic events.

The 1950s and 1960s saw a great number of publications concerning the effects of disruption of affectional bonds. Lorenz (1952) noted that geese and jackdaws separated from their families showed decreased appetite and "acute grief" with the animals seeming to search compulsively for their lost partners. Saul (1962) observed a bitch that became classically depressed for 3 months after the death of the last of her litter. At the end of that time, she showed signs of a spontaneous remission. An interesting reaction has been described in the African parrot which, when exluded from the presence of an observable bond formation, becomes inactive and often dies within 6 months (Dilger, 1960). However, these same African parrots do fine when living in a solitary condition. Only when they must live alone in the presence of an observable bond formation do they have difficulties.

In 1959 Harlow and Zimmerman presented their work with cloth and wire surrogate mothers and their discovery of the development of affectional responses in rhesus monkeys. This classic work has often been keynoted as the beginning of the era of the study of abnormal behavior in primates. Subsequently, many authors began reporting on experimental mother-infant separations or disruption of monkey affectional bonds.

In this chapter I would like to describe first the rationale for animal models and the basic implications of animal models for any form of human psychopathology. Then I will describe two specific approaches to the area of studying depression in young nonhuman primates in order to illustrate the potential value of such work.

One must consider four major areas in developing animal models

(McKinney and Bunney, 1969): (1) induction techniques, (2) documentation of the behavioral syndrome, (3) study of underlying social and/or neurobiological mechanisms, and (4) development of rehabilitation techniques to reverse the syndromes under study.

INDUCTION TECHNIQUES

Induction techniques involve the use of social and/or biological methods to produce a depressive-like syndrome in nonhuman primates. One of the first requirements for an animal model concerns the comparability of inducing techniques across species. Figure 1 illustrates our overall approach to the study of depression in nonhuman primate models, and the general types of induction techniques possible to use can be seen. Of course, one of the big advantages of animal models has to do with the ability to control the inducing techniques systematically so that a certain behavioral syndrome can be associated with a specific inducing event.

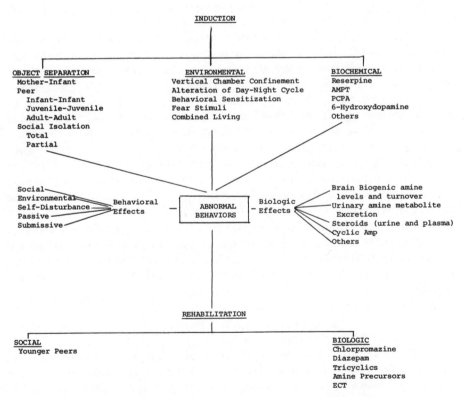

FIG. 1. Experimental psychopathology research approach.

BEHAVIORAL DOCUMENTATION OF THE SYNDROME

Historically, behavioral documentation has been ignored by many investigators. It is not enough to impose a certain inducing condition on an animal, look at the general behaviors, and then say that they represent depression, schizophrenia, autism, etc. Rather, methods must be developed to obtain careful and detailed behavioral profiles on animals that have experienced the various inducing techniques. A number of rating scales are available; they will not be reviewed here, but they involve such things as careful assessment of the frequency of behaviors, the duration of behaviors, the sequencing of behaviors, and the other animals to whom various behaviors are directed along with those animals' responses. The use of trained reliable observers is, of course, essential, and as we will discuss later in this chapter, if both social and biological variables are being studied, exquisite attention must be paid to the development of protocols that will allow assessment of the interacting nature of these factors.

STUDY OF UNDERLYING NEUROBIOLOGICAL MECHANISMS

A major advantage of animal models concerns the ability to study possible underlying neurobiological mechanisms associated with the behavioral syndromes produced without the ethical and practical constraints inherent in human studies. For example, many of the leading neurobiological theories of affective disorders in humans postulate disordered metabolism of one or another brain biogenic amines. However, almost all the evidence for these theories is of necessity indirect. It is not possible to look at the actual brain tissue in depressed humans. The closest studies one can do in this regard involve cerebrospinal fluid studies or brain studies of suicide victims, each of which has its own limitations. On the other hand, in nonhuman primates, a syndrome which is behaviorally similar and similar in terms of the induction technique may allow direct study of brain amine metabolism in relation to the social behaviors exhibited by these subjects. Of special interest would be the study in animal models of neurobiological changes after a social induction technique such as separation in relation to the changes that follow neuropharmacologically induced behavioral alterations. I will illustrate such studies later.

REHABILITATIVE APPROACHES

This work is rather new and involves the development of both social and biological rehabilitative techniques that can be applied to the abnormal animal. Such studies have the potential for helping to clarify the nature of the syndrome produced and for offering improved methods for preclinical evaluation of antidepressants and other drugs. Some work in this area will be illustrated later.

I doubt that I need to caution the reader against the premature use of clinical labels for animal behaviors based strictly on behavioral similarities between species. It is an ethological maxim that two species can arrive at the same final common behaviors from quite different starting points and for quite different reasons, and the behaviors can have quite different significance depending on the context in which they arose. One must be extremely careful in moving from an observable behavior in one species to its application in a different species. I think a considerable amount of prior animal modeling work has suffered from this fallacy.

The remainder of this chapter provides an overview of two differing kinds of induction techniques. The first involves social induction techniques and is based on variations in rearing conditions, and the second approach involves the use of neurobiological techniques to induce abnormal behavior in primates. Then one study is summarized illustrating how primate models can be used to study possible underlying neurobiological mechanisms associated with depression. Finally, our general approaches to rehabilitation of depressed young rhesus monkeys is described in order to illustrate the potential for this approach.

INDUCTION: SOCIAL INDUCTION TECHNIQUES (VARIATIONS IN REARING CONDITIONS)

The two major modifications of rearing conditions that have been used to induce abnormal behavior in primates are social isolation and separation. In my opinion social isolation has less direct relevance to depression, and I will not discuss it in detail. The interested reader is referred to several recent summaries of primate social isolation work, some of which discuss its potential relevance to psychiatric disorders (Harlow et al., 1964; Mitchell and Clark, 1968; McKinney, 1974a).

To set the framework for the section on separation, it should be said that social isolation involves rearing the rhesus macaque for the first 6 to 12 months of life in a situation where no visual, tactile, or other social contact with other monkeys is possible. Isolated rhesus monkeys show deficiencies in behavior that are directly related to the impoverished social environment in which they were reared. When reared for 6 to 12 months in such an environment and then removed and tested socially, they spend the majority of their time engaged in such behaviors as self-mouthing, huddling, rocking, stereotyped behaviors, and marked social withdrawal. Gross deficits are also seen in their aggressive activity, which is inappropriate both in form and in the target of their aggression. As adults they do not engage in appropriate heterosexual behaviors and they are often abusive mothers especially with their first infants.

The severity and persistence of this syndrome is directly related to the amount of time spent in isolation and the age of the rhesus macaque during the isolation period. The most-severe syndrome occurs when the animal is put in isolation at birth and left in for the first year of life. Many clinical terms have been applied to the behavioral manifestations shown by these isolate monkeys and they illustrate several points made in the introduction. Labels such as anxiety, phobia, autism, chronic emotional disorder, behavioral disorder, and experimental neurasthenia have been used too often without adequate behavioral description. This laxity has contributed to the alienation of those clinicians who fail to see similarities between conditions used to produce abnormal behavior in animals and those thought to predispose to human psychopathology. This tendency illustrates that behavioral similarities observable between animals and man do not imply similarities in etiology and significance.

Another social induction technique involves the use of separation experiences; in my opinion, it has more direct relevance to human affective disorders. Often when I am speaking on the topic of animal models, one of the comments frequently made is that the separation work is very interesting but seems mostly relevant to childhood depressions rather than more broadly to adult depression. This is often followed by comments that childhood depressions are quite different and by questions of whether the models are really relevant in a broader sense to affective disorders.

In human children, separation-induced depression has been studied by a number of investigators since Spitz first described the syndrome of anaclitic depression in 1947. Robertson and Bowlby (Robertson and Bowlby, 1952; Robertson, 1955) postulated that the reaction of children and infants to maternal separation occurred in distinct stages. The initial protest stage was characterized by high agitation and attempts to return to the mother. The subsequent despair stage was characterized by weeping and reduced activity. They also described a final detachment phase characterized by withdrawal from any activity and rejection of initial attempts on the part of the mother to reestablish their relationship upon reunion. A number of authors (Jensen and Tolman, 1962; Kaufman and Rosenblum, 1967a; Rosenblum and Kaufman, 1968; Hinde and Spencer-Booth, 1971; McKinney, Suomi, and Harlow, 1972, 1973, 1975; Young et al., 1973; McKinney, 1974b). have reported similar responses in infant rhesus monkeys after separation from their mothers or peers, and this work has suggested the possible existence of behavioral parallels that might provide the beginning for the creation of models of childhood and other forms of human depression.

The above work, however, required the careful description and experimental documentation of the various stages of attachment or "affectional systems" that are important for the developing organism. The affectional systems that have been described in the rhesus monkey include: (1) the infant-mother affectional system; (2) the mother-infant affectional system; (3) the peer affectional system; (4) the heterosexual affectional system; and (5) the paternal affectional system (Harlow and Harlow, 1965). Baseline data were needed in several of the above areas before experimental approaches to the study of separation behavior in young monkeys. Both the normal behavioral characteristics of each of these systems and the sequence in which they mature needed to be described before any scientific understanding of the failure of development of any affectional system or its disruption, once established, could occur. Such data have broadened our perspective concerning developmental processes to include much more than the usual psychodynamic theories.

Laboratory research concerning mother-infant separation in nonhuman primates began with the study of Jensen and Tolman (1962) in which the authors reported results of the separation of two infant pigtail macaques *(Macaca nemestrina)* from their mother for brief periods at 7 and 5 months of age, respectively. Their separation procedure consisted of separating the infants from their mothers, placing them in an observation cage, with either their own or the strange mother, and then reseparating and reuniting with the other mother in the same cage. Thus, their separation was for brief periods and the study was directed toward specificity of mother-infant relationships. The authors reported that in this brief separation-reunion paradigm, the infants and mothers showed high levels of arousal and distress. When the infants were reunited with their own mothers they immediately showed high levels of clinging and similar mother-directed behaviors. However, when reunited with strange mothers, although the infants attempted to establish physical closeness, the strange mothers rejected their attempts. The authors conclude that after brief separation: (1) own infant–directed behavior on the part of the mothers is higher than other infant–directed behaviors; (2) mother-directed behaviors are increased by the infant; (3) learned own-mother specificity occurs after several separations; (4) separation increases the interactive behavior between mother and infant.

Seay, Hansen, and Harlow (1962) studied the effects of separation of four mother-infant pairs. The infants were separated in pairs from their mothers into a common playpen area via a plexiglass panel. Thus, although mother-infant interaction was denied, peer interaction was available during the separation. The authors reported that the infants showed high levels of distress behaviors during the first week of the separation period including increased locomotion, distress vocalizations, and attempts to return to the mother. Throughout the 3-week separation period the infants showed dramatically decreased levels of active play behaviors compared to those seen in the preseparation period. The authors interpret their data as supporting the Bowlby formulation of protest and despair with the exception that the behavior was consistent with Bowlby's description of withdrawal, i.e., detachment was seen only in one of the four infants.

In a similar study, Seay and Harlow (1965) separated two groups of four infants and their mothers in a pen situation wherein the infants had access to each other during 30-min testing sessions daily, although the mothers were removed to another room for the duration of the 2-week separation period. The authors reported an initial protest stage consisting of high levels of locomotion and distress vocalizations. During the period of separation, the level of self-mouthing and social play behaviors decreased, and although the authors do not report the specific time course for the change from increased vocalization-locomotion to "despair" behaviors, they do note such a change. In addition, the authors noted that in contrast to the earlier study where visual contact with the mother was available, in this study where the mother was out of sight and sound, the protest the infants exhibited seemed less intense, although no supporting data are presented for this conclusion.

Hinde, Spencer-Booth, and Bruce (1966) removed the mothers of four infants living in a pen situation for 6 days when the infants were 8 months of age. They found that the infants exhibited a response to the separation similar to that shown by the infants in the studies immediately above: i.e., an initial increase in distress vocalizations and locomotion that persisted for 1 to 2 days. Subsequently, the infants showed lower levels of locomotion and vocalization and a decrease in social and manipulative play throughout the 6-day separation. When the mothers returned, the infants showed higher levels of mother-directed behavior than they had shown in the preseparation period.

Kaufman and Rosenblum (1967b) have studied the effects of mother-infant separation in pigtail macaques. At ages 5 to 6 months, the mothers were removed from the pen situation where the animals had been reared from birth. The separation of the infants took place at different times with some overlap of separations between subjects. The authors reported a clear "agitation" stage lasting 24 to 36 hours in all subjects. This was followed by a "depression" phase lasting an additional 5 to 6 days in 3 of the 4 subjects, and a "recovery" phase lasting through the remainder of the month-long separation in all 4 subjects. Agitation was marked by distress vocalizations, high levels of locomotion, and increased digit sucking. Depression consisted of decreases in activity, increase in huddle, nonlocomotive behavior, and what was subjectively described as the withdrawn characteristics of their behavior. Recovery consisted of lessening of the depression behaviors and increases in more normal patterns of peer play and locomotion. Although the subjective and objective behavioral depression continued, it appeared to be abated. The authors interpreted their data as being consistent with the possible primate model of Spitz's (1946) anaclitic depression and postulated a system of conservation-withdrawal consistent with that of Engel and Reishsman (1956). In contrast to data obtained in the previous study with pigtail macaques, Rosenblum and Kaufman (1968) reported that bonnet macaques (*M. radiata*) subjected to similar separations showed less-severe reactions to separation than did pigtail subjects. They postulate this difference to be owing to basic differences in the social patterns of pigtail bonnet macques. Specifically, bonnets seem to have much higher levels of "passive contact" behaviors than pigtails, and as a result, young bonnet macaques have greater opportunity during early life to form relationships with monkeys other than their own mothers. During the separations the bonnet macaque infants, in fact, established substitute mother-like relationships with other adults when their own mothers were removed. This replacement of the mother-figure perhaps explains why the authors found no behavior corresponding to the depression they found in the pigtail infants.

Spencer-Booth and Hinde (1971) reported the effects of removal for 6 days of the mothers of four 8-month-old infants from stable pen-housed groups of 1 adult male and 4 or 5 adult female rhesus monkeys. They noted that separation was accompanied by increases in vocalizations and a transient increase in locomotion, although locomotion was less vigorous than preseparation locomotion. After the first day, locomotion scores dropped precipitiously to below preseparation levels. The authors describe the change in locomotion along with decreased levels of social interaction and environmental manipulation as being a depression and suggest that their data, although showing no detachment phase, agree with Bowlby's formulation of protest, despair, and detachment responses to maternal separation. In addition, the authors discuss the behaviors of the mother-infant pairs after reunion and note that mother-infant contact increased over preseparation levels with the largest increases being seen in those mother-infant pairs who had highest contact scores before separation.

Spencer-Booth and Hinde (1971) also studied the effects of mother removal for 6 days in 19 rhesus monkey infants when the infants were ages 18, 21, 25, and 30 weeks. They noted that certain of their subjects were separated at two of the ages listed. After comparing data from the various groups, they found that age at separation made no significant difference in the data. They also found that repetition of separation made no difference at a given age. They did find, as in their previous work, that infants at all ages showed depression during the 6 days of separation. They reported no clear increase in locomotion immediately after separation and reported some cases of sharply decreased locomotion. In addition to depression of locomotor activity, the usual suppression of play and environmental manipulation was also found. When mothers and infants were reunited, increased levels of contact were found between mother and infant when compared to preseparation levels. The authors note two caveats, however. First, they found a high degree of variability in the behavior of the infants, and secondly, they cautioned against projecting the meaning of their data onto studies of longer-term separation.

Suomi, Collins, and Harlow (1973) compared the responses of infant rhesus monkeys to permanent separation from their mothers at ages 60, 90, and 120 days. Upon separation, half of the four animals in each group were singly caged while the other two were pair-housed in cages twice as large. The authors found no differences in preseparation behavior in any of the groups. However, responses to separation varied among the various age groups and between pair and singly caged animals after separation. In general, 90-day-old infants showed the severest reaction to separation, and singly housed subjects reacted more intensely than pair-housed subjects. The authors reported more active disturbance in days 1 and 2 than in days 3 through 7 after separation, more passive disturbance in days 1 and 2 than in days 3 through 7, and interactions of both of the above with housing condition and age. Significantly more self-clasp and huddle occurred during days 3 to 7 than in days 1 and 2, and this main effect also interacted with differences of age and housing conditions. Thus, their data roughly fit the protest-despair model of response to mother-infant separation, but in contrast to Spencer-Booth and Hinde (1971), they report differences in response to separation at different ages. The methodologies of the two studies are sufficiently different to contribute to the different findings. Also, Spencer-Booth and Hinde's subjects were on the whole older, 4 to 8 months, as compared to 2 to 6 months in the above study.

In the studies described above, with the exception of the study of bonnet macaques, the response to mother-infant separation roughly fits the classic model of protest and despair, usually occuring within 6 days of separation. However, recent data from the Wisconsin Primate Laboratories, involving five studies of over 20 mother-infant pair separations in the rhesus monkeys at ages 5 to 9 months, do not support a simple protest-despair response model of mother-infant separation (Lewis, 1976). It should be mentioned that this total of 20 rhesus monkeys represents, excluding one study by Hinde and Spencer-Booth (1966), more subjects than previously studied in the entire classic primate separation literature.

It is beyond the scope of this chapter to give the details of each of the five recent studies of mother-infant separation. A few generalizations may be useful for this volume. Data from these studies clearly do not support any unitary concept or an invariant concept of a protest-despair type response to mother-infant separation. The reactions are quite variable and are not predictable enough for maternal separation to be used to provide a useful experimental paradigm for neurobiological and/or rehabilitative studies. This does not mean that maternal separation studies should not be done. Indeed, there is a desperate need for doing such studies to try to ascertain the critical variables in determining the responses of infants to maternal separations. Such studies, both in the human and primate literature, have been neglected for too long and they constitute one of the potential uses of animal models. If there is indeed linkage between separation and depression, both in children and adults, it is important to understand specifically the various parameters of separation. It is difficult to control the interlocking variables in human studies. However, primate studies provide an opportunity to do this and thereby begin to sort out the critical variables in determining response to separation. In a very real sense, this kind of use of primate models has more value than endless debates about whether the behavior shown by a given animal after maternal separation represents "depression," "grief reaction," or other clinical syndromes.

It is clear that consideration of separation paradigms other than maternal separation is necessary to investigate some of the neurobiological mechanisms that might underlie depression as well as possible rehabilitative techniques. Because of this, we are increasingly using peer separation of rhesus macaques as a model for the study of human depression. Work by Bowden and McKinney (1974) and by Suomi, Harlow, and Domek (1970) has suggested peer separation as another useful model. The peer separation model may have a number of advantages. First, the physical act of separating peers is less difficult than separating infants from mothers. Second, the nature of the mother-infant affectional system is normally a rapidly changing one during the first year of life so that age at separation is of critical importance in that paradigm, and large numbers of subjects of identical ages are necessary to generate meaningful data. Third, as an effect of the above, repeated observations in the same subjects of a phenomenon that lasts only a relatively short time is not possible in maternal separation paradigms. Fourth, a consideration of increasing importance is the relatively short period of time that mothers have to be involved in peer separation studies. Current primate resources are for a variety of reasons being limited more and more to within colony production and separation of the infants and their mothers at birth, and subsequent rearing in peer groups means that these mothers are that much more rapidly available for breeding purposes. One can also perform repeated peer separations more easily than repeated maternal separations.

The value of repeated peer separations in this type of work is shown in a recently completed study in which we compared the response to peer separation of rhesus macaques on placebo treatment and on alpha-methyl-para-tyrosine (AMPT) treatment (Morrison, 1976). The details of this study are forthcoming, but in summary we found that AMPT treatment greatly exaggerates the response to peer separation and that there is a significant interaction between drug dosage and response to separation. Also, AMPT has quite different effects when given in a group living situation and when given to monkeys who are separated. This illustrates the potential value of being able to study systematically the social and neurobiological variables that interact to produce a final common pathway to the syndrome of depression.

INDUCTION TECHNIQUES: NEUROBIOLOGICAL METHODS

The basic methodology that we have used involves selective depletion of one or more biogenic amines in the brain combined with observations of resultant behavioral alterations. McKinney et al. (1971) reported the use of reserpine depletion techniques in rhesus monkeys as one means of altering social behavior. At a dosage of 4 mg/kg given daily by intubation for 81 days, significant decreases in locomotion and visual exploration along with increased huddling and posturing were noted. The behavior patterns had many similarities to those seen in the despair stage, which may follow mother-infant or peer separation. However, reserpine is a very nonspecific drug affecting both catecholamines and indoleamines, both in the periphery and in the brain. Subsequent studies have involved the use of alpha-methyl-para-tyrosine (AMPT), para-chlorophenylaniline (PCPA). AMPT at dosages of 250 mg/kg results in behavioral changes quite similar to those seen after reserpine administration, whereas PCPA in dosages up to 800 mg/kg, both in our lab and in the laboratory of Redmond et al. (1971), results in few if any changes in the primates' social behavior.

Because of the peripheral and central effects of both PCPA and AMPT, several investigators have begun to search for more refined methods of studying the relationship between the depletion of brain amines and behavior.

As an example of how primates might be useful in studying depression, we have used 6-hydroxydopamine, which Breese et al. (1970, 1972, 1973) have found to be a selective depletor of central noradrenergic neurons without affecting the serotonergic system or peripheral noradrenergic system. Since central noradrenergic depletions are postulated as a major defect in some forms of human depression, we have continued this work with the goal of experimentally producing this depletion and studying its effects on social behavior and on the pattern of excretion of urinary metabolites after intraventricular administration of 6-hydroxydopamine. Again, the detailed results of this work are beyond the scope of this chapter, but an overview of the approach and of the general results is germaine.

By selective depletion of brain noradrenergic systems in the rhesus monkey, one can indeed produce major alterations in the rhesus monkey's social behavior in the direction of social withdrawal, decreased activity, and decreased levels of arousal. However, the social behavior changes are relatively short-term even though the brain depletions have been shown to be long-term (Kraemer et al., 1975). The possibility of a behavioral compensation even in the face of a continuing brain deficit in the amine system has been suggested, although it is also possible that there is the development of postsynaptic hypersensitivity. It should be mentioned that many of the rhesus monkeys in which this approach has been used are young, that is, 1 to 2 years old, and in a phase of rapidly developing social behaviors.

NEUROBIOLOGICAL MECHANISMS

As an example of this approach one study is summarized which demonstrates that mother-infant separation in rhesus macaques can result in induction of adrenal catecholamine-synthesizing enzymes as well as major elevations in brain serotonin levels (Young, McKinney, Lewis, et al. 1973). In this study, 10 infant rhesus monkeys were reared with their biological mothers in individual living cages. An experimental group of six and a control group of four mother-infant pairs were randomly selected. At 4 months of age, the subjects in the experimental group were separated from their mothers and placed in individual wire cages in another room. During the separation period, the infants could see and hear but not touch each other. Six days after separation from their mothers, the infants were sacrificed. Control animals remained with their mothers until the moment of sacrifice. Behavioral data were obtained for 5 weeks on all animals while they were still housed with their mothers. Observations continued on all animals through the 6 days after the separation of the experimental subjects from their mothers. During the separation period, the experimental subjects showed significant increases in locomotion, environmental exploration, and cooing and screeching vocalization. These responses are typical of the initial protest stage seen after maternal separation. At sacrifice the animals were anaesthetized, the brain removed, and regional dissections done. We also obtained the adrenal glands and the superior cervical ganglia. In those monkeys subjected to separation from their mothers, the adrenal tyrosine hydroxylase level was found to be markedly elevated, as were levels of dopamine β-hydroxylase, phenylethanol N-methyltransferase, and choline acetylase. Catecholamine concentration was not significantly altered. The major significant change in the brain amine levels was an elevation of serotonin in the hypothalamus. Norepinephrine, dopamine, and tyrosine hydroxylase activities in the brains of infant monkeys separated from their mothers were not significantly altered compared with control values in any of the brain regions examined. It is clear from this kind of work that one can, by a social induction technique such as maternal separation, induce major alterations in the peripheral and central brain amine systems. We are continuing our studies to determine comparable findings with animals who are clearly in the despair stage. This approach illustrates another example of the potential usefulness of animal models in studies regarding human depression and separation, which for obvious reasons are not permissible in humans.

REHABILITATION OF ABNORMAL BEHAVIOR IN PRIMATES

We feel strongly that both social and biological techniques should be developed and tried in animal models as well as evaluated for their possible synergistic effects. We have done a series of social and pharmacological rehabilitation studies of socially isolated monkeys. These studies have shown that a severe behavioral syndrome can be altered by pharmacological as well as by social intervention techniques and that therapeutic nihilism is not an appropriate stance (Suomi et al., 1972; McKinney, Davis, and Young, 1973; Noble et al., 1975). The studies have also suggested the social isolation syndrome as a useful model for improved preclinical drug trials.

Of special interest is our recent demonstration that imipramine is effective in reversing the protest-despair response to peer separation as well as modifying the response to future repetitive peer separations. We are currently evaluating other agents in both the peer separation paradigm as well as the social isolation syndrome.

Obviously one has to be especially careful in reasoning from such drug rehabilitation studies. The fact that a peer separation protest-despair reaction is reversed by imipramine does not in itself "prove" that the syndrome under question necessarily represents depression. These kinds of data must be viewed as one piece of the puzzle in relation to other criteria such as comparability of inducing conditions, behavioral similarities, and underlying neurobiological mechanisms. A variety of other agents of different classes must also be tried if we are to understand fully the significance of the initial imipramine data.

CONCLUSIONS

I feel that our work, as well as the work of others in different laboratories, has by now clearly demonstrated that the study of animal models can have relevance for our understanding of depression in the young developing organism. The development of criteria by which to evaluate models and the study of the interaction between social and biological variables in such models have been two major breakthroughs. It should be remembered, however, that this field is new, with the modern era representing only approximately 8 to 10 years. This is indeed young for a research field, and a considerable amount of additional work is in order. In the near future, research with animal models directed toward understanding of the neurobiological mechanisms underlying the separation reaction is particularly important. The behavioral consequences of manipulation of the biogenic amine systems at various developmental stages has considerable potential relevance for a better understanding of childhood depression. Also of importance is careful behavioral observation so that one can eventually define better the behavioral aspects of the syndrome recognized as depression. One of the future tasks with regard to animal model work concerns the controlled study of differing kinds of variables interacting with each other as illustrated by the conjoint use of separation techniques and AMPT administration. Close collaboration between clinicians and animal researchers is important as a sense of trust and mutual understanding must continue to develop between these two groups in order to facilitate progress in the application of animal models for the better understanding of childhood depression and other forms of mental disorders.

ACKNOWLEDGMENTS

The writing of this paper and the research reported were supported by Research Grant # MH 21892 and by Research Scientist Career Development

Award # MH 47353, both from the National Institute of Mental Health, and by the Wisconsin Psychiatric Research Institute.

REFERENCES

Bowden, D. M., and McKinney, W. T. Effects of selective frontal lobe lesions in response to separation of adolescent rhesus monkeys. *Brain Res.*, 75:167–171, 1974.

Breese, G. R., and Traylor, T. C. Effect of 6-hydroxydopamine on brain norepinephrine and dopamine: Evidence of selective degeneration of calecholamine neurons. *J. Pharmacol. Exp. Ther.*, 174:413–420, 1970.

Breese, G. R., Cooper, B. R., and Smith, R. D. Biochemical and behavioral alterations following 6-hydroxydopamine administration into brain. In E. Usdin and S. Snyder (eds.): *Frontiers in Catecholamine Research: Third International Catecholamine Symposium.* New York, Pergamon Press, 1973.

Breese, G. R., Prange, A. J., Howard, J. L., Lipton, M. A., McKinney, W. T., Bowman, R. E., and Bushnell, P. 3-Methoxy-4-hydroxyphenylglycol excretion and behavioral changes in rat and monkey after central sympathectomy with 6-hydroxydopamine. *Nature [New Biol.]*, 240:286–287, 1972.

Dilger, W. C. The comparative ethology of the African parrot genus agapornis. *Z. Tierpsychol.*, 17:649–685, 1960.

Engel, G. L., and Reishsman, F. Spontaneous and experimentally induced depressions in an infant with gastric fistula: A contribution to the problem of depression. *J. Am. Psychoanal. Assoc.*, 4:428–452, 1956.

Harlow, H. F., and Harlow, M. K. The affectional systems. In A. M. Schrier, H. F. Harlow, and F. Stollnitz (eds.): *Behavior of Nonhuman Primates*, New York, Academic Press, 1965.

Harlow, H. F., and Suomi, S. J. Induced psychopathology in monkeys. *Engineering Sci.*, 33:8–14, 1970.

Harlow, H. F., and Zimmerman, R. R. Affectional responses in the infant monkey. *Science*, 130:421–432, 1959.

Harlow, H. F., Rowland, G. L., and Griffin, G. A. The effect of total social deprivation on the development of monkey behavior. In P. Solomon, and B. C. Gluech (eds.): *Psychiatric Research Report IV.* Washington, D.C., American Psychiatric Association, 1964.

Hinde, R. A., Spencer-Booth, Y., and Bruce, M. Effects of 6-day maternal deprivation on rhesus monkey infants. *Nature*, 210:1021–1023, 1966.

Hinde, R. A., and Spencer-Booth, Y. Effects of brief separation from mother on rhesus monkeys. *Science*, 173:111–118, 1971.

Jensen, G. D., and Tolman, C. W. Mother-infant relationship in the monkey, Macaca nemestrina: The effect of brief separation and mother-infant specificity. *J. Comp. Physiol. Psychol.*, 55:131–136, 1962.

Kaufman, I. C., and Rosenblum, L. A. Depression in infant monkeys separated from their mothers. *Science*, 155:1030–1031, 1967a.

Kaufman, I. C., and Rosenblum, L. A. The reaction to separation in infant monkeys: Anaclitic depression and conservation-withdrawal. *Psychom. Med.*, 29:648–675, 1967b.

Kraemer, G. W., McKinney, W. T., Breese, G. R., Howard, J. L., and Prange, A. J. Effects of 6-hydroxydopamine in the rhesus monkey. Presented at the American Psychiatric Association, 1975.

Kubie, L. A. The experimental induction of neurotic reactions in man. *Yale J. Biol. Med.*, 11:541–545, 1939.

Lewis, J. K., McKinney, W. T., Jr., Young, L. D., and Kraemer, G. W. Mother-infant separation in rhesus monkeys as a model of human depression. *Arch. Gen. Psychiatry*, 33:699–705, 1976.

Lorenz, K. Z., *King Solomon's Ring*, New York, Thomas Cornwell Co., 1952.

McKinney, W. T. Animal models of psychiatry. *Perspect. Biol. Med.*, 17:529–541, 1974a.

McKinney, W. T. Primate social isolation: Psychiatric implications. *Arch. Gen. Psychiatry*, 31:422–426, 1974b.

McKinney, W. T., and Bunney, W. F. Animal model of depression. I. review of evidence: Implications for research. *Arch. Gen. Psychiatry*, 21:240, 1969.

McKinney, W. T., Davis, J. M., and Young, L. Chlorpromazine rehabilitation of disturbed monkeys. *Arch. Gen. Psychiatry,* 29:490–494, 1973.

McKinney, W. T., Eising, R., Moran, E., Suomi, S. J., and Harlow, H. F. Effects of reserpine on the social behavior of rhesus monkeys. *Dis. Nerv. Syst.,* 32:735–741, 1971.

McKinney, W. T., Suomi, S. J., and Harlow, H. F. Repetitive peer separations of juvenile age rhesus monkeys. *Arch. Gen. Psychiatry,* 27:200, 1972.

McKinney, W. T., Suomi, S. J., and Harlow, H. F. New models of separation and depression in rhesus monkeys. *Separation and Depression: Research Aspects,* pp. 53–66, 1973.

McKinney, W. T., Suomi, S. J., and Harlow, H. F. Experimental psychopathology in non-human primates. In D. Hamburg (ed.): *American Handbook of Psychiatry.* New York, Basic Books, 1975.

Mitchell, G. D., and Clark, D. L. Long term effects of social isolation in nonsocially adapted rhesus monkeys. *J. Genet. Psychol.,* 113:117–128, 1968.

Morrison, H. L. Protest—despair response to peer separation in rhesus monkey and its potentiation by alteration of calecholamine metabolism. Presented to American Psychosomatic Society, Pittsburg, 1976.

Noble, A. B., McKinney, W. T., Mohr, C. A., and Moran, E. C. Diazepam treatment of socially isolated monkeys. Presented at the American Psychiatric Association, 1975.

Premack, D. A. A functional analysis of language. *J. Exp. Anal. Behav.,* 14:107–125, 1970.

Redmond, D. E., Maas, J. W., Kling, A., Graham, C. W., and Dekirmenjan, H. Social behavior of monkeys selectively depleted of monoamines. *Science,* 174:428–431, 1971.

Robertson, J. Some response of young children to loss of maternal care. *Nurs. Times,* 49:382–386, 1955.

Robertson, J., and Bowlby, J. Responses of young children to separation from their mothers. *Cour du Centre International de l'Enfance,* 2:131–142, 1952.

Rosenblum, L. A., and Kaufman, I. C. Variations in infant development and response to maternal loss in monkeys. *Am. J. Orthopsychiatry,* 38:418–426, 1968.

Saul, L. J. Psychosocial medicine and observation of animals. *Psychosom. Med.,* 24:58–61, 1962.

Seay, B., and Harlow, H. F. Maternal separation in the rhesus monkey. *J. Nerv. Ment. Dis.,* 140:434–441, 1965.

Seay, B., Hansen, E. W., and Harlow, H. F. Mother-infant separation in monkeys. *J. Child Psychol. Psychiatry,* 3:123–132, 1962.

Seligman, M. E. Fall into helplessness. *Psychol. Today,* 7:43–48, 1973.

Seligman, M. E., and Maier, S. F. Failure to escape traumatic shock. *J. Exp. Psychol.,* 74:1–9, 1967.

Senay, E. C. Toward an animal model of depression: A study of separation behavior in dogs. *J. Psychiatr. Res.,* 4:65–71, 1966.

Spencer-Booth, Y., and Hinde, R. A. The effects of separating rhesus monkeys from their mothers for 6 days. *J. Child Psychol. Psychiatry,* 7:179–197, 1967.

Spencer-Booth, Y., and Hinde, R. A. The effects of 13 days maternal separation on infant rhesus monkeys compared with those of shorter and repeated separation. *Anim. Behav.,* 19:595–605, 1971.

Spitz, R. A. Anaclitic depression: An inquiry into the genesis of psychiatric conditions in early childhood. II. *Psychoanal. Study Child,* 2:313–342, 1947.

Suomi, S. J., Collins, M., and Harlow, H. F. Effect of permanent separation from mother on infant monkey. *Dev. Psychol.,* 9:376–384, 1973.

Suomi, S. J., Harlow, H. F., and Domek, C. J. Effect of repetitive infant separation of young monkeys. *J. Abnorm. Psychol.,* 76:161–172, 1970.

Suomi, S. J., Harlow, H. F., and McKinney, W. T. Monkey psychiatrists. *Am. J. Psychiatry,* 128:927, 1972.

Young, L., McKinney, W. T., Lewis, J. L., Breese, G. R., Smith, R. D., Mueller, R. A., Howard, J. L., Prange, A. J., and Lipton, M. A. Induction of adrenal catecholamine synthesizing enzymes following mother-infant separation. *Nature,* 246:94–96, 1973.

Young, L., Suomi, S. J., Harlow, H. F., and McKinney, W. T. Early stress and later response to separation. *Am. J. Psychiatry,* 130:400–405, 1973.

Depression in Childhood: Diagnosis, Treatment, and Conceptual Models, edited by J. G. Schulterbrandt and A. Raskin. Raven Press, New York, 1977.

Depression and the Perception of Control in Early Childhood

John S. Watson

Department of Psychology, University of California, Berkeley, California 94720

Within the past decade there has arisen an impressive array of evidence which identifies a rather simple experiential variable as a fundamental cause of depression. In both animals and humans, depression appears to be the direct consequence of exposure to significant events that are outside the subject's control. It can be argued that the most basic adaptive capacity of animate life is the ability to alter behavior in the service of either increasing or decreasing one's probable contact with biologically significant events. It now would seem that when this capacity is thwarted by contrived experiences in a laboratory or by extraordinary experiences in the real world, most animals and humans enter a pathological state of diminished behavioral initiative and emotional disturbance, a pathological state encompassing if not all that is implied by the general term "depression," then at least much of that implied by the common variety termed "reactive depression" (Seligman, 1975).

In a recent review of the evidence for this causal relationship between uncontrollable stimulation and depression, Seligman (1975, p. 99) came to the following conclusion: "To the degree that uncontrollable events occur, either traumatic or positive, depression will be predisposed and ego strength undermined. To the degree that controllable events occur, a sense of mastery and resistance to depression will result."

Three objectives are set for this chapter. First, it provides a brief review of the experimental research that has focused on the effects of exposure to stimulation independent of a subject's behavior, commonly termed "noncontingent stimulation." In the context of Seligman's recent extensive survey of this literature (Seligman, 1975), the present review is limited to the historically more salient of the previous research and to some research with human infants that has been conducted since the time of Seligman's review. A point to be emphasized by this chapter and illustrated in particular by the recent infant data is that positive stimulation, because of its great invasive potential, deserves perhaps even more serious attention than aversive stimulation as a general causative factor in the etiology of childhood depression.

The second objective of this chapter is to consider some of the theoretical implications of recent research as regards the basic environmental and organismic variables involved in a child's perception of control. Although the concept of control is rather simple and the effects of its absence seem to be clear, it is not at all clear just what determines the perception of controllability. It seems a safe assumption that controllable events whose control is imperceptible will have the same effects as events that are, in fact, uncontrollable. If one accepts this assumption, then it is obvious that a full understanding of the circumstances leading to depression in childhood will require an understanding of the variables that contribute to the perception of control in childhood.

The third objective of the chapter is to outline the questions that appear most in need of research in this area. On the basis of the preceding review and theoretical analysis, experimental and observational lines of investigation are suggested.

RESEARCH ON THE EFFECTS OF NONCONTINGENT STIMULATION

In the existing literature on the effects of exposure to stimulation not contingent on behavior, the earliest and most common investigations are those that have involved escape from, or avoidance of, aversive stimulation. In one of the first of this variety of studies (McCulloch and Bruner, 1939), rats subjected to 1,000 sec of unavoidable shocks were later trained on a forced-choice brightness discrimination problem with shock as punishment for errors. These rats made more errors than did controls that had not been previously subjected to shock. Data presently available indicate that the diminished instrumental discrimination of the shocked rats was not an effect of receiving shock *per se* but rather of receiving unavoidable shock (i.e., not contingent on any behavior). Furthermore, although this early study relies on errors of behavior to index a failure of the *covert* act of discrimination, studies since have demonstrated failure to initiate instrumental activity with *overt* behavior. These more recent studies extend beyond the rat (e.g., Anderson, Schwendiman, Taylor, and Peckham, 1967; Anderson, Cole, and McVaugh, 1968; Maier, 1972) to animals as diverse as the dog (Overmier and Leaf, 1965; Overmier and Seligman, 1967; Seligman and Maier, 1967), the goldfish (Behrend and Bitterman, 1963; Pinckney, 1967), and the cockroach (Herridge, 1962; Pritchatt, 1968).

Perhaps the most provocative overt behavioral evidence of the effect of noncontingent aversive stimulation on the later initiation of instrumental activity was presented in a series of reports from a research group at the University of Pennsylvania (e.g., Maier, Seligman, and Solomon, 1969; Seligman, Maier, and Solomon, 1971). In an incisive series of experiments with dogs, these researchers made a number of interesting discoveries about the onset and development of what they called the "interference effect." They have also offered a theoretical concept, "learned helplessness," to account for the effect (Maier, Seligman, and Solomon, 1969; Seligman, 1975).

A dramatic display of the interference effect was observed by this research group in a two-way shuttlebox in which avoidance of shock by the dog required jumping over a hurdle dividing the box in two sections within 10 sec of the onset warning signal. If the dog jumped the hurdle, the warning signal terminated without shock. If the dog failed to jump the hurdle, the warning signal remained on and was accompanied by shock for up to 50 sec or until the dog jumped to safety. Naive dogs performed strikingly differently from dogs that had been subjected to 64 unsignaled, inescapable shocks 24 hr before entry into the shuttlebox. Seligman, Maier, and Solomon (1971) reported that over a series of studies, "Sixty-three percent of dogs pretreated with inescapable shock fail to escape on 9 out of 10 trials (N = 82), while only six percent of naive animals fail (N = 35)." Their description (p. 11) of the reaction of the dogs to the situation was impressive:

The behavior of the preshocked dogs was bizarre. When they got the first shock in the shuttlebox, they looked like the naive dogs: They frantically ran about, howled, defecated and urinated. However, unlike naive dogs, they soon stopped running around and quietly whimpered until the trial terminated. They seemed to 'give up' and passively 'accept' shock. On succeeding trials, these dogs continued to fail to make escape movements. A few dogs would get up and jump the barrier, escaping or avoiding shock, yet, surprisingly, on the next trial such a dog would go back to taking shock. It did not seem to learn that barrier-jumping produced shock termination.

The developmental course of this interference effect with dogs was found to have two important temporal features. First, the effect depends on the experience of uncontrollable shocks preceding any experience in which the shocks are controllable. If the animal is first given an opportunity to control shock and then experiences uncontrollable shock, the interference effect does not occur. Second, the effect wanes, becoming undetectable after 48 hr. Yet if a dog experiences unavoidable shocks and then fails to learn to control contingent shock 24 hr later, it will be incapable of learning to avoid shocks for up to a month. Thus, vast individual differences between dogs can be produced as a function of the timing of just one experience with uncontrollable shock.

After reviewing all their data, Seligman, Maier, and Solomon (1971) concluded that this interference effect in dogs could not be adequately explained by appeal to concepts of "adaptation" or "sensitization" to shocks, "competing motor responses," or "emotional exhaustion." They offered "learned helplessness" as the best single explanation. The concept is a significant extension of the concept of "helplessness" introduced by Mowrer and Viek (1948) as a potential basis of fear arousal. That a sense of helplessness may lead to fear and its concomitants is surely important. But the fact that a learned sense of helplessness may deactivate the initiation of instrumental responding is even more important in a consideration of adaptive functioning in general and depression in particular. As applied to the interference effect of experiencing uncontrollable shock, the learned helplessness model was described by its authors (Seligman, Maier, and Solomon, 1971, pp. 31–32) as follows:

(1) Subject (S) makes active responses during exposure to inescapable shocks.

(2) Because shock cannot be controlled, S learns that shock termination is independent of its behavior.

(3) S's incentive for initiating active instrumental responses during shock is assumed to be partially reduced by its *expectation* that the probability of shock termination will be increased by these responses. When this expectation is absent S should have little incentive for active instrumental attempts.

(4) The presence of shock in the escape/avoidance training situation should then arouse the same expectation that was previously acquired during exposure to inescapable shock: shock is uncontrollable. Therefore, the incentive for initiating and maintaining active instrumental responses in the training situation should be low.

Seligman (1975) has argued forcefully that this learned helplessness model is no less applicable to man than to dogs or other lower animals. He has reviewed the experimental and clinical evidence for the interference effects of noncontingent aversive stimulation in humans. Although it is not ethically possible to generate experimental data that would parallel the animal experiments, the studies that have been carried out with mildly aversive stimulation do generally support the learned helplessness model. Seligman also reported impressive clinical evidence that supports the contention that humans are subject to the interference effect. This clinical evidence has led him to two notable extensions of the general model. One extension is that the interference effect may occur in fewer trials as the significance of the noncontingent event increases. Perhaps even a single event such as the death of a loved one would be sufficient. In effect, this is a one-trial learning proposal for the learned helplessness model. The second extension is of at least equal significance. Seligman proposes that the interference effect of perceiving that one has no control over significant events may be so strong as to not only eliminate adaptive instrumental initiative but even to undermine life-supporting behaviors (e.g., heartbeat) as well. With these extensions of the original model, it is not surprising that Seligman is willing to propose that the clinical syndrome of depression can be viewed as a severe form of the interference effect. Thus, from this perspective the perception of having no control is no longer viewed as a symptom of depression but rather as its most fundamental cause.

Now it is important to note that the interference effect, whether minimal or massive, is an effect of perceiving the lack of control which derives from experiencing an event that is not dependent on one's behavior. This is in contrast to *lack* of experience with an event that is dependent on one's behavior. The important experiential variable is assumed to be the occurrence of aversive stimulation, regardless of when or what behavior preceded it.

Experiencing the absence of aversive stimulation regardless of when or what behavior preceded it does not seem very important for understanding the experimental evidence inasmuch as a naive subject could be expected to have massive amounts of this null experience before the avoidance training situation. Although this distinction between the occurrence of nothing and the nonoccurrence of something may at first appear merely academic (if not whimsically philosophical), the distinction is necessary for understanding the relationship between the interference effects of noncontingent aversive stimulation and those of noncontingent positive stimulation. We shall return to this distinction after considering the research on positive stimulation.

STUDIES WITH POSITIVE STIMULATION

Comparatively few studies have involved an analysis of the effects of an initial experience with noncontingent positive stimulation on later performance in a situation in which the stimulation is contingent on behavior. These studies have been primarily with young humans (e.g., O'Brien, 1969; Watson, 1971; Millar, 1972; Finkelstein and Ramey, 1975; Foster and Vietze, 1975), although there have been a few reports from work with rats and pigeons (e.g., Seligman, Meyer, and Testa, 1971; Engberg, Hansen, Walker, and Thomas, 1973). Overall, the limited data available on both covert and overt responses are highly consistent with those obtained with aversive stimulation.

O'Brien (1969) examined the effect on nursery school children of experiencing the receipt of reward (candy) noncontingently before performance on a discrimination learning task. While sorting three-dimensional forms in a game situation, the experimental subjects initially received reward in a pattern unrelated to the manner in which they sorted the forms. Control groups either received no reward in this initial situation or received it in a manner that was contingent on the way in which they sorted the forms. All subjects later received the reward contingent on the "correctness" of their sorting behavior. Subjects who had initially received noncontingent reward learned less well than either control group. Thus, as was observed with the manipulation of aversive stimulation by McCulloch and Bruner (1939), the covert act of discrimination appears to be less probable if the stimulation rewarding it has previously been experienced noncontingently.

Overt instrumental activity has also been observed to be disengaged by noncontingent positive stimulation. Watson (1971) reported a study showing this effect on head movements in infants. Beginning at 8 weeks of age, infants received a 10-min exposure to a mobile each day for 2 weeks in their homes. The mobile turned periodically in a manner unrelated to their behavior. Other infants were exposed either to a mobile that remained stationary for the 10-min exposure or to a mobile that turned contingent on head movement. At 10 weeks of age the infants all had an opportunity to control the mobile with head movements in a laboratory setting. Infants who had experienced either no turning or contingent turning in their homes increased their head movements significantly in the laboratory setting when the mobile turning was contingent. However, those infants who had viewed the mobile turning noncontingently for 2 weeks showed no increase in head movement. Six weeks later, with no exposure to the mobile in the interim, all infants were again examined in the laboratory setting. The results were the same, indicating that the effect of noncontingent exposure could last up to 1½ months for infants who were only 2 months old when they received the noncontingent stimulation.

Interestingly, Millar (1972), also working with human infants, found that exposure to noncontingent presentation of an audiovisual stimulus before its use as a reinforcement for arm movement led to an increase in the learning rate during later response-contingent presentation of the stimulus. It is notable, however, that Millar's experiment involved only 1 session with a total of 3 min of exposure to noncontingent stimulation, whereas Watson's experiment involved 14 sessions with a total of 140 min of exposure. This contrast suggests the likely possibility of there being an inverted-U relationship between noncontingent exposure and the reinforcement potency of a stimulus. Positive "predifferentiation" effects have been found in animals and children for discriminative stimuli (Gibson, 1969). It seems a reasonable assumption that the perception of control depends to some extent on the discriminability of the stimulus. If that is so, then the question immediately arises as to when noncontingent exposure stops improving the reinforcement potency of a stimulus through predifferentiation and begins decreasing the potency through the growing effect of interference. One might well expect that this turning point will vary as a function of the particular stimulus and as a function of the species and age of the subject. A recent report by Foster and Vietze (1975) indicates that noncontingent exposure of the mobile stimulus to human infants begins to show interference effects after approximately 6 min of presentation.

Overall, then, the major parallel in findings for positive and aversive stimulation is clear. The eventual failure to initiate instrumental activity appears to be a consequence of experiencing an event that is not dependent on behavior as opposed to being a consequence of a lack of experience with an event dependent on behavior. Usually we expect the absence of a positive event to function similarly to the presentation of a negative one and the lack of a negative event to function similarly to presentation of a positive one. But in the case of the interference effect, positive and aversive events appear to have the same function rather than the opposite.

The practical importance of this basic similarity is great. It means that the interference effect can arise in the context of events we would normally describe as benevolent as well as in those we would describe as malevolent. It implies that parents might lead their young toward depression by actions and deeds we otherwise would view as open (noncontingent) expressions of affection. Moreover, one can imagine that the general rate of noncontingent positive stimulation might rise sharply within the child-rearing practices of a society with much less notice than would accrue to an equal increment in the general rate of noncontingent aversive stimulation.

This latter point is illustrated by some data gathered in the author's laboratory during the past year. A study of 8-week-old infants learning to control a mobile with head movement was carried out in a follow-up of the Foster and Vietze (1975) study of short-term noncontingent exposure. The single-session laboratory experiment involved a 10-min learning period that was preceded by a 10-min exposure to the mobile turning noncontingently for half of the 32 subjects. To our dismay, however, neither the group with nor the group without prior noncontingent stimulation showed any general learning. Examination of interview records with the mothers of the infants revealed that more than 60% of these infants were presently being exposed to at least one automatic "wind-up" mobile at home. The usual variety of this wind-up mobile turns while playing a nursery tune for approximately 5 min after being wound. Similar interview data available from a study carried out 6 years previously showed that only 12% of our samples ($N = 48$) were then being exposed to this automatic mobile. Since the old and new samples were at the same age and from the same social class and geographic locale, the contrast implies a very significant shift upward ($\chi^2 = 21.92$; $p < 0.001$) in at least one form of noncontingent stimulation in the child-rearing practices of the San Francisco Bay Area middle class.

Of equal interest to this sharp rise in exposure to commercially produced automatic mobiles was the result of a *post hoc* analysis of learning records, which indicated that those infants who obtained high individual learning scores (as assessed by rate change in the contingent period) either had no automatic mobile or, if they had one, also were described by their mothers as having gained control (by kicking or batting) of some toy hanging over their crib.

We recognized that this implication of an interference effect from the home being responsible for obscuring an interference effect in the laboratory was much too convenient to be trusted. Another study was carried out specifically to follow-up this finding. Forty-nine 14-week-olds were presented with a single learning session in which foot movement controlled a mobile turning and a bell tone. A learning score was derived for each infant based on the change in response rate from the last of the 3 min of a preliminary base period to the last of the following 9 min of response contingency. The infants were independently classified in four groups based on interview data relating to exposure to automatic mobiles at home and to display of control over any hanging toy in their crib. The results clearly corroborated the *post hoc* findings of the previous study. The mean learning scores for the four subgroups were each positive except for the subgroup exposed to an automatic mobile and who did not display control of any hanging toy at home ($N = 11$). This group showed an unreliable yet notable decline in response rate. The only subgroup to display statistically reliable learning as evidenced by a rise in response rate was that in which the infants had not been exposed to an automatic mobile and had also displayed some control over a hanging toy at home ($N = 9$; $t = 2.51$; $p < 0.05$). On the basis of an index of response differentiation obtained by observing the correlation of foot and head movement, this subgroup was also the only group to display a significant differentiation of behavior (a shift from $r = 0.68$ to -0.03 from the 3rd min of the base period to the 9th min of the contingency· period).

It would seem, then, that the recent rise in exposure to noncontingent stimulation has not been without consequence for these infants. Whether our measures of learning are all that have been affected or whether this interference effect has a wider range of transfer for these infants is not yet known, although Finkelstein and Ramey (1975) report transfer of interference to a novel response and reward with 6-month-old infants. The case illustrates well the potential invasive possibilities for interference effects from positive noncontingent stimulation. It seems unlikely that a similarly effective rise in noncontingent aversive stimulation could have occurred without having also stirred considerable social alarm.

PERCEPTION OF CONTROL

Before concluding this review of the learned helplessness or interference model of depression, it would be useful to consider at least briefly what is presently understood about the process commonly referred to as perception of control. When an event occurs it may or may not be contingent on one's behavior. Clearly, a basic assumption of the helplessness model is that interference effects follow when the subject fails to perceive a contingency between his behavior and the event. However, surprisingly little is known about the conditions that govern whether or not a controllable event is perceived as controllable. Of course, the interference effect itself is an instance of apparently misperceiving an existing contingency. The assumption of the learned helplessness model is that this misperception is derived as a generalization from prior perception of noncontingency. But what governs the accuracy of perception in the formative experience?

One approach to this question is to ask what environmental variables might be expected to "mask" an existing contingency and what organismic factors might be expected to affect an individual's acuity in the perception of behavioral efficacy. The vast literature on learning suggests many candidates, of course. Such environmental variables as a delay between behavior and consequence (delayed reinforcement), a less-than-perfect contingency (partial reinforcement), and poor signaling of contingency availability (lack of discriminative stimuli) would be expected to reduce the clarity of a contingency. Likewise, the organismic factors of lower memory capacities to span delays (short term) and recognize recurrences (long term) of limited or inappropriate attentional functions and of poor response rate (producing dysfunctional distribution of practice) would be expected to affect adversely the likelihood that an existing contingency would be accurately perceived. Clearly, we have no paucity of candidates from the general learning literature. Nevertheless, virtually no information is available on how these masking factors work individually or interactively to produce interference effects in either the laboratory or the real world.

As a case in point, consider what little is understood of this perceptual problem in human infancy. On the basis of existing research, it would appear that an existing contingency can be effectively masked within the first 6 months of life if the delay of effect is as short as 3 sec (Ramey and Ourth, 1971; Millar, 1972), if the rate of behavior does not provide recurrences within at least 7 sec (Watson, 1967), or if the probability of reward is not nearly perfect (Watson, 1975). To the extent that these findings can be generalized beyond their laboratory origins, it seems amazing that the human infant ever perceives any contingencies in the real world. Are most events, then, perceived as uncontrollable during early infancy? If that were so, the learned helplessness model should predict massive interferences and susceptibility to depression as normal products of human infancy. In the face of this unlikely prospect, one might assume that the interference effects of perceiving uncontrollability are to some extent dependent on prior experience of perceiving control. But there is no experimental evidence for this hypothesis of "you can't miss it till you've had it."

The point of this chapter is not to cast doubt on the learned helplessness model of depression. Rather, it is to emphasize the central role played in this theory by "perception of control" and to point out the severe limitations of our present understanding of this process variable.

IMPLICATIONS FOR RESEARCH

If one accepts the assumption that much of what is clinically termed depression can be viewed as the real world workings of the interference effect (Seligman, 1975), then it is obvious that much further research of both the experimental and observational varieties will be needed. From an experimental standpoint, much more work is needed on factors influencing the perception of control as was pointed out above. In addition, studies of the generalization characteristics of interference effects are needed. Will positive noncontingent stimulation lead to helplessness in a subsequent context of aversive events? How important are intensity and diversity of stimulation? How easily can discriminative control be established? Answers to these questions would have relevance to theories of both etiology and therapy. Eventually, one would hope that sufficient information would be available to justify experiments on preventative and therapeutic intervention in the development of depression in children.

Observational studies are also needed. Particularly useful would be studies that can inform us of the timing characteristics of contingent and noncontingent stimulation during childhood. The frequency, intensity, and diversity of both positive and aversive stimulation would also be ecological variables of relevance. Comparing normal and "at risk" samples on these variables could provide a powerful real world evaluation of the interference model of depression. Finally, given the invasive potential of noncontingent positive stimulation, relevant observation should be made of possible transitions in child-rearing conditions through time.

ACKNOWLEDGMENTS

The studies reported here from the author's recent research were supported by Grant MH 24283-01 from the National Institute of Mental Health. Thanks are extended to Mrs. Melissa Lagusis, Mrs. Allyson Rickard, Mrs. Carol George, and Mr. Richard Ewy for their assistance in the collection and analysis of data.

REFERENCES

Anderson, D. C., Cole, J., and McVaugh, W. Variations in unsignalled, inescapable preshock as determinants of responses to punishment. *J. Comp. Physiol. Psychol. (Monogr. Suppl.,* Part 2), 65:1–17, 1968.

Anderson, D. C., Schwendiman, G., Taylor, J., and Peckham, S. Does inescapable unsignaled preshock always produce conditioned apathy? Read at annual meeting of the Western Psychological Association, 1967.

Behrend, E. R., and Bitterman, M. E. Sidman avoidance in the fish. *J. Exp. Anal. Behav.,* 13:229–242, 1963.

Engberg, L. A., Hansen, G., Walker, R. L., and Thomas, D. W. Acquisition of key-pecking via autoshaping as a function of prior experience: "learned laziness"? *Science,* 178:1002–1004, 1973.

Finkelstein, N. W., and Ramey, C. T. Learning to control the environment in infancy. Read at Biennial Meeting of Society for Research in Child Development, 1975.

Foster, M., and Vietze, P. The role of visual attention to non-contingent stimulation in predicting later learning with three-month-olds. Read at Biennial Meeting of Society for Research in Child Development, 1975.

Gibson, E. J. *Principles of Perceptual Learning and Development.* New York, Appleton-Century-Crofts, 1969.

Herridge, G. A. Learning of leg position by the ventral nerve cord in headless insects. *Proc. R. Soc. Biol.,* 157:33–52, 1962.

Maier, S. F. Helplessness: current animal studies. Read in Symposium on Helplessness at Annual Meeting of American Psychological Association, 1972.

Maier, S. F., Seligman, M. E. P., and Solomon, R. L. Pavlovian fear conditioning and learned helplessness. In B. A. Campbell and R. M. Church (eds.): *Punishment.* New York, Appleton-Century-Crofts, pp. 299–343, 1969.

McCulloch, T. L., and Bruner, J. S. The effect of electric shock upon subsequent learning in the rat. *J. Psychol.,* 7:333–336, 1939.

Millar, W. S. A study of operant conditioning under delayed reinforcement in early infancy. *Monogr. Soc. Res. Child Dev.,* 37(2), 1972.

Mowrer, O. H., and Viek, P. An experimental analogue of fear from a sense of helplessness. *J. Abnorm. Soc. Psychol.,* 43:193–200, 1948.

O'Brien, R. A. Positive and negative sets in two-choice discrimination learning by children. Master's thesis, Urbana, University of Illinois, 1969.

Overmier, J. B., and Leaf, R. Effects of discriminative Pavlovian fear conditioning upon previously or subsequently acquired avoidance responding. *J. Comp. Physiol. Psychol.,* 60:213–217, 1965.

Overmier, J. B., and Seligman, M. E. P. Effects of inescapable shock upon subsequent escape and avoidance responding. *J. Comp. Physiol. Psychol.,* 63:28–33, 1967.

Pinckney, G. Avoidance learning in fish as a function of prior fear conditioning. *Psychol. Rep.,* 20:21–74, 1967.

Pritchatt, D. Avoidance of electric shock by the cockroach periplaneta americana. *Anim. Behav.,* 16:178–185, 1968.

Ramey, C. T., and Ourth, L. L. Delayed reinforcement and vocalization rates of infants. *Child Devel.,* 42:291–297, 1971.

Seligman, M. E. P. *Helplessness: On Depression, Development and Death.* San Francisco, W. H. Freeman, 1975.

Seligman, M. E. P., and Maier, S. F. Failure to escape traumatic shock. *J. Exp. Psychol.,* 74:1–9, 1967.

Seligman, M. E. P., Maier, S. F., and Solomon, R. L. Unpredictable and uncontrollable aversive events. In F. R. Brush (ed.): *Aversive Conditioning and Learning.* New York, Academic Press, pp. 347–400, 1971 (page references in text are to prepublication mimeographed copy of manuscript distributed in 1970).

Seligman, M. E. P., Meyer, B., and Testa, T. Appetitive helplessness: Non-contingent reinforcement retards instrumental learning. Unpublished manuscript, University of Pennsylvania, 1971, cited by Seligman (1975).

Watson, J. S. Memory and "contingency analysis" in infant learning. *Merrill-Palmer Q.,* 13:55–76, 1967.

Watson, J. S. Cognitive-perceptual development in infancy: Setting for the seventies. *Merrill-Palmer Q.,* 17:139–152, 1971.

Watson, J. S. Can partial reinforcement explain behavioral persistence in infants? Read at Biennial Meeting of Society for Research in Child Development, 1975.

Learned Helplessness: A Developmental Approach

Discussion of the Chapters by Drs. McKinney and Watson

Carol S. Dweck

Department of Psychology, University of Illinois, Champaign, Illinois 61820

A discussant at this point is in the somewhat unenviable position of evaluating the applicability of the learned helplessness model to a phenomenon that might not exist—childhood depression. Be that as it may, I will outline the issues and offer a contingency plan.

The major question thus far has been: Is there such an entity as childhood depression that is equivalent or analogous to the syndrome that has been identified in adults? If there is, then the question for the present purposes becomes whether the learned helplessness model provides a useful way of conceptualizing its etiology, its characteristics, or its treatment. If there is no such entity, one would wish to identify the nature of the chief mood disorders that children *do* experience (those that have been labeled "depression") and to determine whether learned helplessness is useful in understanding and perhaps alleviating these disorders. In addition, one might ask whether learned helplessness in childhood can serve as a predictor of depression in adulthood.

If it is found that true depression does exist in childhood, then the arguments that Seligman (1975) has advanced to support the learned helplessness analysis of adult depression are applicable and I would refer the interested individual to his excellent book. If, on the other hand, depression is not found to exist in children in a form that bears enough resemblance to the adult syndrome to warrant the same label, then helplessness is still likely to be applicable to the kinds of mood disorders that make up a major part of children's emotional problems.

It is most intriguing, however, to consider the possibility that learned helplessness in childhood is the precursor of depression in adulthood. That possibility constitutes the focus of this chapter. It is proposed that: (1) learned helplessness in childhood may lead to depression in adulthood even though childhood disorders have not been found to predict adult depression; (2)

concluding that depression does not occur before adolescence does not argue for the primacy of biochemical over psychological causes; and, (3) the learned helplessness analysis is not incompatible with the absence of depression in childhood, even though children have less control over their environments than do adults.

LEARNED HELPLESSNESS: DEFINITION AND BACKGROUND

First, let us specify what learned helplessness is and is not. It refers to the *perception* of independence between one's responses and the onset or termination of aversive events. That is, from the person's point of view, the probability of avoiding or escaping a noxious event is the same whether he responds or not. It should be noted that this definition does not imply that a helpless individual necessarily perceives aversive events as noncontingent or unrelated to his behavior. On the contrary, an individual can view aversive events as being a direct consequence of his behavior, but he is helpless to the extent that the aversive situation is seen as insurmountable; i.e., the probability of altering the undesirable state of affairs is not affected by any response the individual feels he is capable of performing. Thus, the helpless individual views the occurrence of an aversive event as a signal that he cannot control the situation and often as a cue for the continued occurrence of such events despite efforts on his part.

Our own work with children in achievement situations (e.g., Dweck and Reppucci, 1973; Dweck, 1975) has demonstrated the striking consequences of such cognitions. We have investigated children's differing reactions to failure experiences as a function of their causal cognitions. Helpless children are those who tend to attribute failures to factors that are beyond their control, such as external agents or their own lack of ability. Nonhelpless children tend to see failures as owing to easily modifiable aspects of their behavior, such as their lack of effort. The helpless children are in all cases every bit as competent at problem-solving as the nonhelpless children—before failure. Once failure occurs, however, their behavior rapidly disintegrates to the point that they are no longer capable of solving the very problems they had solved with ease only shortly before. In short, they become passive, demoralized, and essentially incompetent in the face of failure. The nonhelpless children, in contrast, show improved performance when they are confronted with failure. They tend to vary their behavior systematically and use failure as a cue to devise alternative strategies for tackling the problem. Only when the learned helpless children are taught to attribute their failures to factors they can control do they begin to confront failures in a more active and successful manner. Thus the quality of children's coping responses in the face of aversive events is a function not of their ability to perform the requisite behavior, but rather of the causes to which they attribute those events and the implication of these attributions for their future outcomes.

LEARNED HELPLESSNESS AS A PREDICTOR OF ADULT DEPRESSION

How can helplessness simultaneously explain childhood disorders that *are not* depression and predict disorders that *are* depression when, as Drs. Gittelman and Lefkowitz point out, childhood disorders are not found to predict adult depression? That is, how can one assert that helplessness is at the base of early mood disorders and later ones when the two are statistically unrelated? This apparent contradiction may be resolved by assuming, first, that not all helpless children will display problematic behavior. As our own studies suggest, helpless children are as competent as others until they encounter adversity, at which point their instrumental responses deteriorate severely. Many of these children encounter no adversity of sufficient magnitude in childhood for these patterns of cognitions to pose a serious obstacle to their adjustment. Second, of those helpless children who do evidence problems in childhood, some are helped to cope successfully whereas others are not. One would predict adult disorders to be less likely for those who have had experiences that allow them to learn that negative environmental events are controllable. Those who do not cope will be candidates for adult mood disorder. Finally, those who are not helpless in childhood may be unlikely to become so as adults. These possibilities are depicted in Table 1. Thus helplessness may be conceptualized as necessary but not sufficient for serious mood disorders. The critical variable, then, may be the degree to which childhood experiences have taught one to view aversive events as surmountable.

If depression is found not to exist before adolescence, then one might argue against the learned helplessness model in either of the following ways.

1. Finding that depression does not occur before adolescence argues for the primacy of biochemistry. That is, a physiologically mature organism is necessary for the biochemical disruptions that cause depression.

2. If perceptions of inability to control outcomes produce depression, then why aren't children more prone to depression than adults? After all, it is they who have, in some absolute sense, less control over their environment than do adults.

However, in adolescence, when the physiological-maturational changes are

TABLE 1. *Proposed likelihood of postadolescent depression as a function of preadolescent learned helplessness, emotional disorders, and coping*

Preadolescence		Postadolescence
Helpless — No disorder		Depression
— Disorder — Coping		No depression
— No coping		Depression
Nonhelpless		No depression

taking place, two important psychological and social changes are also occurring:

1. In the adolescent period the child is entering a new stage of cognitive development—the period of formal operations. At this time abstract, hypothetical thought becomes possible. Before this time the child is able to ponder and to manipulate cognitively only entities that have a concrete reality, and he cannot extrapolate his experiences to all possible situations. During the period of formal operations, however, the child becomes capable of questioning, for example, the meaning of life, and of reflecting on its ultimate worth—in short, of having an "identity crisis." Helpless cognitions, once triggered, can become generalized to all possible realms and for all possible times, leading to the perception of generalized, perpetual hopelessness.

2. In order for failure to exert control to have alarming implications for the individual, it must occur in the face of a necessity to exert control or an expectation of control. Only then does failure have important consequences for one's future or for one's competence. Nearing adolescence the child is expected to assume an adult role. He then experiences increasing pressure from adults and peers to take responsibility for his outcomes and exert control over his environment.

Thus, learned helplessness may not result in true depression before adolescence because the necessity for control and expectations that one exert control are not as great as they are later in life, and the possible cognitive and emotional consequences of lack of control are not as far-reaching. However, the tendency to react to adversity with helpless cognitions, combined with a lack of experience in encountering and coping with adversity, may predispose an individual to depression in the postadolescent period—despite the absence of apparent problems earlier in life.

To argue in favor of the role of cognitions in depression is not to argue against the role of biochemistry. It would be foolish to deny the profound effects that alterations in biochemistry can have on mood and cognition. There are undoubtedly important individual differences (and intraindividual differences over time) in biochemistry that influence one's susceptibility to helpless cognitions and depression after aversive events. However, there are also likely to be individual differences in the ease with which aversive events will trigger helpless cognitions, which in turn will trigger biochemical changes. The learned helplessness model may provide a way of understanding the role of childhood experiences in the development of such differences.

REFERENCES

Dweck, C. S. The role of expectations and attributions in the alleviation of learned helplessness. *J. Pers. Soc. Psychol.,* 31:674–685, 1975.

Dweck, C. S., and Reppucci, N. D. Learned helplessness and reinforcement responsibility in children. *J. Pers. Soc. Psychol.,* 25:109–116, 1973.

Seligman, M. E. P. *Helplessness: On Depression, Development, and Death.* San Francisco, W. H. Freeman, 1975.

Overview and Future Directions

Depression in Childhood: Diagnosis, Treatment, and Conceptual Models, edited by J. G. Schulterbrandt and A. Raskin. Raven Press, New York, 1977.

Depression in Children: Fact or Fallacy?

Allen Raskin

Psychopharmacology Research Branch, National Institute of Mental Health, Rockville, Maryland 20857

A major preoccupation of contributors to this volume has been the definition or diagnosis of depression in children. Some investigators felt the adult diagnostic model as described by Feighner and his associates (1972) and later adapted by Spitzer, Endicott, and Robins (1974) in their *Research Diagnostic Criteria (unpublished manuscript)* could be applied to children. Basically, this was the approach adopted by investigators who served on the Subcommittee on Clinical Criteria for the Diagnosis of Childhood Depression. To be diagnosed as depressed, a child had to manifest dysphoric mood plus additional associated symptoms including evidence of anhedonia or a loss of interest in "previously pleasurable activities." An additional criterion imposed by this group was a minimum of 4 weeks duration of these symptoms and behaviors.

Subsequent discussion of these recommendations by the contributors revealed that comparatively few children currently being seen in in- or outpatient mental health facilities would meet these criteria. In particular, it was felt that the requirement of 4 weeks of essentially umremitting depression would rule out many children in whom depression was an especially frequent but not a constant mood state.

The definition and/or diagnosis of depression in children was also complicated by a number of developmental, epidemiological, and psychosocial factors. Dr. Lefkowitz noted in his discussion of Dr. Gittelman's chapter that many of the signs or symptoms usually associated with depression in children or adults, such as fears and worries, occurred with surprisingly high frequency in a random household sample of children in Buffalo, New York (Lapouse and Monk, 1958; Lapouse, 1966). This study also revealed that the incidence of these "deviant" behaviors was age related with an excess of high scores among the 6- to 8-year-old group as compared with the 9- to 12-year-old group. These results raised serious questions regarding the meaning one should attach to these apparent behavior deviations, namely, as Lapouse and Monk remarked, are they "truly indicative of psychiatric disorder or . . . (do) they occur as transient developmental phenomena in essentially normal children."

A related problem evident in this volume was concern over the reference group or groups to use for purposes of sampling or rating depression in children. This issue has its counterpart in the adult depression literature as well with efforts to distinguish depression as a syndrome, or symptom cluster associated with a specific diagnostic group, from depression as a symptom. Depressive symptoms can occur in association with grief reactions such as the death of a loved one or can be the normal accompaniments to physical illness such as cancer or severe burns. Dr. Gittelman developed this point in her chapter and distinguished four subgroups of children with depressive symptomatology. She described a group with primary or endogenous depression, another with situational dysphorias, and two groups with depression as an accompaniment of other behavioral disorders. Other investigators raised similar questions with regard to the presence of depressive symptoms in children subjected to frequent and irrational beatings (the battered child), children who continually experience failure in school because of dyslexia or hyperactivity, and even children with nutritional deficiencies who may mimic the anergia and listlessness seen in some depressed children and adults.

A major practical concern of the authors with regard to these issues was the possible misuse of drugs, such as the antidepressant drug imipramine, to treat children in whom depression was a more or less normal accompaniment of situational factors, such as child abuse, and would dissipate if the outside source of the depression were removed. Conversely, some authors felt there may be a group of endogenously depressed youngsters who are generally not easily recognized or identified and who might benefit from exposure to an antidepressant such as imipramine. These latter children may also constitute a group at high risk for later adult depression and share a predisposition to depression with their parents or siblings on the basis of similar genetic or biochemical factors. We are certainly becoming more aware and interested in both genetic and biochemical predispositions to depression in adults, and it would be logical to extend these interests to children as well. Consequently, the need to identify accurately the incidence and prevalence of depressive symptomatology in children and to distinguish among children with endogenous as distinct from situational depression is not only of academic interest but has important practical implications for both treatment and prognosis.

Although at times contributors to this volume despaired of ever resolving these issues, research strategies for dealing with these issues did eventually emerge and are included in a number of the chapters and discussion sections. Having these chapters and discussions available puts me in an enviable position. I would like to take advantage of this opportunity by borrowing ideas from the other authors and adding a few of my own in an effort to combine the approaches of the various investigators into a coordinated research plan for defining depression in children.

First, some consensus is needed on the critical behaviors that constitute the signs or symptoms of depression in children. Drs. Kovacs and Beck are willing to finesse this issue temporarily by starting with behaviors which they admit have traditionally been used to describe depression in adults rather than in children. The children's version of the Beck Depression Inventory (BDI), which Drs. Kovacs and Beck have labeled the Children's Depression Inventory (CDI), taps essentially the same basic dimensions of depression present in the BDI but one inappropriate item has been omitted and the wording has been simplified to make the individual items more understandable to young children. Pilot work with this scale on a small sample of 7 children, ages 9 to 15, in a child guidance center, showed wide variability in total CDI scores, which suggested the scale might have predictive validity in distinguishing depressed from nondepressed youngsters.

Although Drs. Kovacs and Beck were able to demonstrate considerable overlap between items that authors have used to describe depression in children and items that have proven useful in this regard in adults, I am not sure one should eliminate entirely from the scale those behaviors generally cited under the rubric of "masked depression" because these behaviors are often difficult to interpret and do not provide a direct measure of depression in children. Generally, the behaviors used to characterize masked depression in children are hostile or aggressive in tone and include temper tantrums, disobedience, running away from home, delinquency, and truancy. It is not uncommon in the adult depression literature today to find reference to the presence of both depression and outward expressions of hostility in the same individual despite the psychoanalytic dictum that in depression hostility is repressed and directed inward and therefore fails to find adequate expression in behavior. Consequently, the complete absence of items that tap feelings of hostility and resentment on the CDI may be a serious omission at this stage of our knowledge regarding the critical behaviors that characterize childhood depression. If there is, in fact, a subgroup of hostile-depressed children, they would probably be overlooked if ratings were limited to the CDI.

As a strategy for developing an instrument or instruments for measuring depression in children, I also feel there are some obvious advantages in starting with a fairly long laundry list of symptoms and behaviors which different authors have reported to be associated with depression in children. In Tables 1 and 2 of the chapter by Kovacs and Beck, there is considerable overlap in the behaviors cited by the various authors as characterizing childhood depression. Consequently, a 35- to 50-item symptom checklist could be constructed that would incorporate 90% of the various items listed in these two tables.

An additional issue is the choice of rater. Although the CDI is completed by a test examiner, it was also my impression that the child specifically is asked to respond to the CDI items and is essentially the prime source for completion of the items. Experience with adult depression rating scales suggests that the child is probably the best source for reporting or rating his inner feeling states but may not be an especially reliable source for rating such things as appetite and sleep disturbances, expressions of hostility, loss of pleasure in activities previously enjoyed, etc. The child's parents, teachers, or in the case of hospitalized youngsters, the ward nurses may be better sources for rating the presence of these secondary symptoms of depression. At this exploratory stage it would probably be best to think of developing simultaneously three or four separate rating instruments, one based essentially on information obtained directly from the child, one completed by the child's parent(s), one completed by the ward nurse, and possibly a fourth completed by a teacher. Although there may be some overlap in the items sampled by each of these rating instruments, the laundry list of signs and symptoms of depression referred to earlier would be assigned to the rating instrument and rating source that has the best opportunity to observe and sample the behavior in question.

Reference was previously made to the variability of children's mood states, which can fluctuate from day to day or even from hour to hour. This variability may also be more pronounced in younger (7 to 9) than in older (10 to 12) children. It may therefore make sense to separate those symptoms and behaviors that are likely to show dramatic changes, such as mood items, and to rate these more frequently than items that generally persist for more extended periods, such as appetite disturbances and loss of interest in activities previously enjoyed.

Let us assume we have followed the steps previously outlined and now have a mood scale designed to be completed jointly by the child and a test examiner on a daily basis, a symptom checklist that a psychiatrist or psychologist can complete weekly, and a behavior inventory that the parent and/or teacher can also complete on a weekly basis. We must now face what is undoubtedly the most troublesome and perplexing problem in this field, namely, how do we find or select the depressed youngsters to validate these scales. A possible starting point would be to find children in circumstances where it would be reasonable to assume that they must be experiencing some feelings of despair and depression. Children who have recently experienced the death of a parent, children with chronic failure experiences in school, battered children, children with physical illnesses that require long periods of hospitalization, and children who have recently witnessed the dissolution of their parents' marriage would all seem logical candidates for an initial validation of the items on childhood depression scales. For comparative purposes it would also be necessary to administer these scales to "normal" youngsters to identify those scale items which best discriminate the presumed depressed child from the normal matched child of the same age, sex, IQ, and social class background. If these scales are later to be used in establishing norms or cutoff scores for distinguishing normal from pathological depression, it will probably be necessary to sample selectively by age group (e.g., 7 to 9 versus 10 to 12), sex, social class, and intelligence. Prior reference was made to the finding that behaviors deemed deviant in older children occurred with high frequency and therefore appeared normal when found in younger children. Similar findings may emerge when the relationships between depression in children and social class status, sex, and intelligence are examined.

If we have been successful in establishing the criterion-oriented validity of these scales in the sense that the scale items retained for use do significantly differentiate the high-risk for depression children from normal children, we are ready to test these scales on children admitted to in- and outpatient mental health facilities. Our aims at this stage of the research will be twofold. First, we wish to see if these scales retain their validity by discerning signs and symptoms of depression in children admitted to these mental health facilities. Second, we are interested in the utility of these scales as diagnostic tools in identifying subgroups of depressed children. Hopefully, these subgroups will later prove to be clinically distinguishable in terms of the presumed etiology of their depression, response to treatment, and prognosis.

To achieve the second aim it will be necessary to have some preconceived conceptual or theoretical bases for selecting children from the mental health facilities for inclusion in the study. In other words, if we posit, as Dr. Gittelman has done, that there are four distinct subgroups of depressed children, then we should be certain that we have sampled adequately to bring representative children from each of these subgroups into the study. This issue would be especially critical with regard to the so-called masked depressions where the major focus would be on behaviors not usually associated with depression. It will also be necessary to obtain from family informants social and psychiatric history data such as a history of depression or psychiatric illness in parents or siblings, some data on life stress events, measures of social adjustment at home and in school, and indications of possible lifelong neuroticism. Measures of school adjustment and acting-out behavior should also be obtained. The criteria for including children in the study at this stage should be relatively liberal. Children who are obviously schizophrenic, autistic, or psychopathic and who show no apparent evidence of depression would be excluded. On the other hand, if the clinician suspects that a child's delinquency, truancy, or somatic complaints are associated with some underlying depression, the child should be admitted. Children with dysphoric mood would also be admitted even if this mood state were of relatively short duration, e.g., 2 weeks, and subject to considerable variability from week to week. To avoid overinclusion of atypical childhood depressions, researchers should admit to the sample sufficient numbers of depressed children who meet the criteria enunciated by the Subcommittee on Clinical Criteria for the Diagnosis of Childhood Depression (see page II).

After the children have been rated on the symptom and behavior rating scales, some data reduction techniques, such as deriving composite or super factors of psychopathology, may be in order before efforts are made to identify homogeneous clusters or subgroups of children. The statistical techniques that come to mind for the latter purpose are cluster analysis or inverse factor analysis. To obtain meaningful clusters or groups of children, it would be necessary to include in these analyses not only the symptom data but selected information from the social and psychiatric history forms as marker variables. A history of depression in the mother is an example of an important marker variable that may be associated with a specific pattern of symptoms. An additional marker variable of some importance would be a measure of the persistence of the depression in the child. A small group of endogenously depressed children may have periods of depression lasting 1 month or longer. However, other groups of depressed children may be considerably more variable in this regard.

In summary, I have outlined procedures one might use to arrive at empirically derived subtypes of depressed children. As I noted earlier, many of these procedures were suggested by other contributors to this volume. Obviously, it is not possible to predict in advance what the outcome of such a research strategy or proposal might be. At the very least, it would provide some normative data on the incidence of certain signs and symptoms of depression both in normal children and in high-risk groups such as battered children which would be useful in their own right. At best, we may end up with meaningful subgroups of depressed children that could have important implications for both treatment and prognosis.

The title of this chapter asks if depression in children is a real or fancied phenomenon. I am sure nobody questions that children are both capable of experiencing depression and do, in fact, become depressed. The unresolved issues are how children express or manifest depression; how pervasive, intense, and long-lasting these feelings and associated behaviors are; and whether there are subgroupings of depressed children with differing etiologies, patterns of symptoms, responses to treatment, and susceptibility for later adult depression. It seems to me that we should be asking these questions rather than the more general question of whether depression exists in children. Also as outlined in this chapter, these questions are researchable and lend themselves to empirical investigation.

REFERENCES

Feighner, J. P., Robins, E., Guze, S. B., Woodruff, R. A., Winokur, G., and Munoz, R. Diagnostic criteria for use in psychiatric research. *Arch. Gen. Psychiatry,* 26:57–63, 1972.

Lapouse, R. The epidemiology of behavior disorders in children. *Am. J. Dis. Child.,* 111:594–599, 1966.

Lapouse, R., and Monk, M. A. An epidemiologic study of behavior characteristics in children. *Am. J. Public Health,* 48:1134–1144, 1958.

Depression in Childhood: Diagnosis, Treatment, and Conceptual Models, edited by J. G. Schulterbrandt and A. Raskin. Raven Press, New York, 1977.

Epilogue: Future Considerations and Directions

Stephen P. Hersh

National Institute of Mental Health, Rockville, Maryland 20014

At this time, neither our social nor our health care system recognizes the existence of depression in the prepubescent child. One expression of this nonrecognition is the fact that in most county, state, and national data systems, one cannot identify anyone under 17 years of age carrying either the depression or affective disorder label. Another expression of nonrecognition is that most psychology and psychiatry texts either fail to refer to depression in childhood or, if they do refer to it, do so only in regard to very special situations such as marasmus, adjustment reactions to parental divorce, or acute injury or illness.

Today the public recognizes depression and many of its consequences in the older teenager and the adult. Much of this recognition stems from research efforts over the past 30 years. Perhaps our cultural mythology is responsible for the nonrecognition of depression in children. That mythology sketches childhood as the age of innocence, of no responsibilities, of play and happiness. It allows us to see children as at times sulking or being moody or mad, bad, or glad, but for the most part they are to be joyful.

To my mind, the immediate challenge is to learn more about the origins and evolution of affective states in the human. Such studies in the ontogeny of mood disorders should probably begin with the fetus. It is in the context of such investigations that questions concerning depressive illness and depressive equivalents will be articulated and most responsibly answered.

Dimensions to investigate include biology, the environment, and the interaction of the two. Studies in the biological dimension include work by T. Berry Brazelton and his colleagues (*personal communication* and Brazelton, 1976) at Children's Hospital in Boston, revealing the possibility that some human newborns may have a reduced capacity to relate to and elicit relatedness from adult caring figures. Also in the biological dimension are studies by Gordon Bronson (1968, 1972*a,b,* 1976) of Mills College, Oakland, California, which indicate that a significant minority of first-year infants are temperamentally disposed toward heightened wariness (a tendency to stop activity, pout, cry, or avoid new situations), and that this unusual tendency towards wariness during infancy may be, for that 20% of newborns, a precursor to the development of relatively enduring social unease. There are recent psycho-physiological studies by individuals such as Joseph Campos (1975*a,b;* 1976*a,b*) of the University of Denver, showing that various experience states have different effects on different infants in terms of the responses of the autonomic nervous system. Indeed, there are studies that show the existence of some children with apparent poor regulatory ability of the autonomic nervous system. These children have fitful, restless sleep and appetite distur-bance. One wonders how or whether such children differ from others in their mood responses to stress. A few children who are given the minimum brain dysfunction label and treated with amphetamines show, as a side effect to the medication, a behavioral response similar to that seen in the withdrawn adult depressive syndrome (Rapoport, 1976).

Studies of environmental impact should include investigation of training received from parent figures in mastery and nonmastery. Studies are also needed concerning the long-term impact of life experiences and the many, often dramatic, alterations in mood which they produce with children.

Interactions between biology and environment help form the psychological and psychosocial dimensions of an individual. Whereas the same life experi-ences may produce the same mood responses in different people they do not produce the same mood disorders. The Kovacs/Beck pilot studies as well as the Lefkowitz data indicate that mood disorders involving sadness, poor self image, and mood motivation may be very common in the general child population; indeed, such mood disorders may be a basic affective element of the growth and development of children. Research strategies can be varied and may include treatment studies, genetic/familial studies, behavioral studies of signs and symptoms, and studies of function and response to stress. One can design studies using a definition based on clinical experience, such as James Anthony's definition concerning the inability to express pleasure. One can begin, as Kovacs and Beck suggest, by using the adult model of depres-sion to describe different relatively stable mood states, and examine their antecedents and natural course as well as their responses to psychopharma-cological agents. In examining the natural history of such mood states, one can also, as with adult affective disorders, examine genetic backgrounds.

In summary then, studies in the development of affective states in infants and children are called for. Such studies will not only lead to a greater understanding of dysphoric states, of mood disorders, but will significantly enrich our understanding of the adult depressive syndrome: its history, course, and response to treatment. For despite the impressive development over the last 10 years, work on adult depression is not as precise as imagined and never will be until the ontogeny of affective states is better understood.

REFERENCES

Brazelton, T. B. Early parent-infant reciprocity. In V. C. Vaughan and T. B. Brazelton (eds.): *The Family—Can It Be Saved?* Chicago, Year Book Medical Publication, pp. 133–142, 1976.

Bronson, G. W. The development of fear in man and other animals. *Child Dev.,* 39:409–431, 1968.

Bronson, G. W. Fear of the unfamiliar in human infants. In H. Schaffer (ed.): *The Origins of Human Social Relations.* London, Academic Press, 1972a.

Bronson, G. W. Infants' reactions to Unfamiliar Persons and Novel Objects. *Monographs of the Society for Research in Child Development,* 37 (3, Serial No. 148), 1972b.

Bronson, G. W. On the distinction between wariness and fear, 1976 (*in preparation*).

Campos, J., Emde, R., Gaensbauer, T., and Henderson, C. Cardiac and behavioral interrelationships in the reactions of infants to strangers. *Developmental Psychol.,* 11:589–601, 1975a.

Campos, J. The operational definition of "fear" and recent studies of "fear of strangers." Educational Retrieval Information Center (ERIC), Baltimore, University of Maryland, 1975b (*in press*).

Campos, J. Heart rate: A sensitive tool for the study of emotional development. In L. Lipsitt (ed.): *Psychobiology: The Significance of Infancy.* Washington, D.C., Larry Erlbaum Associates, 1976a (*in press*).

Campos, J. Thesis, antithesis, and synthesis: Freedman's implications for the future of the nature-nurture conflict. In L. Lipsitt (ed.): *Psychobiology: The Significance of Infancy.* Washington, D.C., Larry Erlbaum Associates, 1976b (*in press*).

Rapoport, J. L. Psychopharmacology of childhood depression. In Donald Kline and Rachel Gittelman Klein (eds.): *Progress in Psychiatric Drug Treatment, Vol. 2,* New York, Brunner Mazel, 1976.

Appendix:
Areas for Research and Development

Depression in Childhood: Diagnosis, Treatment, and Conceptual Models, edited by J. G. Schulterbrandt and A. Raskin. Raven Press, New York, 1977.

Summary of the Subcommittee on Clinical Criteria for Diagnosis of Depression in Children

Carol S. Dweck, Rachel Gittelman-Klein, William T. McKinney, and John S. Watson

The following criteria were arrived at for a diagnosis of depression in children: Both items 1 and 2 are necessary.

ESSENTIAL CLINICAL FEATURES

1. Dysphoria.
2. Generalized impairment in response to previously reinforcing experiences, without the concomitant introduction of new sources of reinforcement. This impairment is manifested by a reduction in instrumental, self-initiated activities across broad classes of behavior. Previously pleasurable activities are no longer effective in regulating behavior.

The above has to be generalized across settings and not be specific to isolated areas of functioning.

Associated Features

Characteristics of dysphoria and reduced response to reinforcements are probably associated with different secondary symptoms at various ages. Empirical investigations are necessary to determine what aspects of behavior and cognitive function are altered at various developmental levels. These would consist of changes in self-esteem, guilt (i.e., notions of personal responsibility), personal and general pessimisim (i.e., negative expectations about oneself or life in general), or blaming others.

DURATION

A minimum duration of 4 weeks is stipulated for the diagnosis to be made.

SOURCES OF INFORMATION

Interview observations and reports by significant others would be necessary for the determination of the clinical syndrome. No single source of information would be deemed adequate for a formulation of the diagnosis.

It was felt that the NIMH needs to develop incentives for research career grants in child psychiatry so that systematic investigations of depressive disorders and other childhood disorders may be generated. At present, there is no pool of child psychiatrists sophisticated in research procedures to ensure the generation of data so lacking in childhood behavior disorders.

Depression in Childhood: Diagnosis, Treatment, and Conceptual Models, edited by J. G. Schulterbrandt and A. Raskin. Raven Press, New York, 1977.

Conclusions and Recommendations of the Subcommittee on Assessment*

Maria Kovacs, Chairperson

INTRODUCTION

At the present time, the psychopathology of childhood depression is an exceedingly difficult area to investigate. There is lack of descriptive agreement on the constituents of the phenomenon. Assessment and formal diagnostic tools are sorely lacking. Some people question the very existence of depression in childhood.

The development of descriptive agreement and viable assessment procedures is hindered by lack of data on normal developmental variations in mood and associated behaviors. Finally, dramatic differences in cognitive and behavioral repertoires at various ages in childhood mediate against a uniform approach toward early depressive pathology.

The committee's recommendations on the assessment of early childhood depressions are made within the limitations imposed by the above factors. As one step toward a viable set of recommendations, the committee found it expedient to agree on the following assumptions:

1. Depression as a clinical picture is a syndrome.
2. The depressive syndrome presumably results or manifests in observable or measurable impairment in functioning.
3. The syndrome necessitates different assessment approaches in "younger" as opposed to "older" children.
4. Description and assessment of clinical phenomena go hand in hand.

The notion that description and assessment are difficult to separate was especially evident in the committee's discussions. As some members pointed out, the choice of measurement instruments tends to define the phenomenon under consideration. Moreover, descriptive agreement (e.g., diagnosis) has been traditionally one of the criteria used to validate clinical assessment tools.

---

*Members: C. Keith Connors, Carl P. Malmquist; Observers: Allen Raskin, Ben Locke.

Consequently, the committee recommended strategies that may lead to descriptive agreement of childhood depressions and discussed viable approaches in the area of assessment. As a possible direction for future research, the committee also formulated a few general research questions that may help explore description and assessment of childhood depressions.

The committee also felt that there are at least two basic, crucial questions that investigations should seek to answer: (1) What number of symptoms, or severity of symptoms, is sufficient criterion to justify the diagnosis of childhood depressive syndrome; and (2) What is the duration of symptoms necessary for a "clinical syndrome" diagnosis?

RECOMMENDED STRATEGIES FOR DESCRIBING THE PHENOMENOLOGY OF CHILDHOOD DEPRESSIONS

The committee members felt that the following general research strategies may be useful in yielding clinical agreement on the characteristics of childhood depressions.

Strategy A. Start with the working hypothesis that the symptoms of adult depression exist in childhood. Assess the validity of this hypothesis with special reference to duration and transience of the syndrome in children.

Strategy B. Through a systematic survey of adults who work with children (e.g., clinicians, pediatricians, teachers, parents, child welfare case workers), elicit descriptions of childhood depression. Reduce the resulting data to a list of core and auxiliary symptoms.

Strategy C. Define the problem as the systematic description of grief reactions at different ages: list the number, type, and duration of symptoms for each age group. Examination of large populations of children who have lost a parent or a parent substitute may facilitate a description of clinical depression as a statistically deviant response to loss.

Strategy D. Study "index" children, who, based on *a priori* definitions, can be expected to manifest current or future symptoms of depression. The index children may be "high-risk" children defined in terms of a genetically biased population or in terms of having a clinically depressed parent.

The third strategy outlined above was strongly favored by the committee. The members felt that strategy C may be profitably used to address the following issues: (1) "normal" (± 1 SD) duration of dysphoria and other symptoms in view of objectively defined loss; (2) extent and type of associated behavioral impairments; (3) invariance of the symptoms as a function of exposure to different situations; (4) developmental variations in the syndrome as a function of age; and (5) actual prevalence of the syndrome.

Given a large enough population, it may be assumed that the various characteristics will be normally distributed. Thus "normal" grief reactions may be distinguished from "clinical" depressive reactions based on statistical infrequency of occurrence.

RECOMMENDATIONS ON THE ASSESSMENT OF CHILDHOOD DEPRESSIONS

Discussion concerning the assessment of childhood depressions is summarized under the following headings: measurement instruments, raters, sampling problems, and study designs.

A problematic dimension that underlies all the above categories is the subjects' age range. The committee arbitrarily defined "younger" children as children aged 7 or below and "older" children as those aged 8 and above. This age cutoff was based on the extent of verbal-conceptual abilities and the development of reading comprehension in school-aged youngsters above the 2nd grade, which increase the possibility of reliable self-reporting and the use of written tests.

Measurement Instruments

In view of all the problems outlined in the introduction, the committee felt that the measurement of childhood depressions is best undertaken through a multifaceted, multibattery approach.

Some committee members felt that in such a test battery both the data-gathering approaches and the content of the instruments should be varied.

It was recommended that the *content* of the measurement instruments cover the areas listed below; the format of the instruments (e.g., multiple choice, true-or-false, open ended, item ranking) may be decided by content appropriateness and expediency:

1. *Facial expression and motoric behavior.* At the time of the interview, facial expression of affect and gross motoric retardation or agitation should be rated.

2. *Social responsivity–social adjustment.* The current patterning of social responses as well as apparent disruptions of previously patterned responses should be rated. Social responsivity pertains to the way in which the child relates to:

   a. parents (responding to affection, age-related social demands in the family),

   b. peers (characteristics and/or changes in the quality and quantity of play activity), and,

   c. teachers (responses to school-related cooperative and task demands).

3. *Task performance.* Ratings of task performance should focus on the child's ability to be involved in, undertake, and execute age-related tasks. Current performance should be evaluated in light of previous performance level or generally accepted age norms. For example, disruptions in previously patterned self-grooming activities may be assessed. Other worthwhile tasks to be focused on may

include homework performance, picking up after oneself, obtaining things for oneself, etc.

4. *Problem-solving strategies.* Another content area worthwhile to investigate is the child's strategies for solving problems. The problems should be relevant to the child's world, e.g., problems of being punished, being made fun of, not being paid attention to, not having one's way, being ignored/neglected. The strategies may be assessed under:

  a. affective strategies (sadness, crying, anger, blandness, resentment, anxiety),

  b. behavioral strategies (yelling, fighting, destroying, crying, withdrawal-silence),

  c. cognitive strategies (feeling bad about oneself, blaming others, feeling "no good," unworthy).

5. *Concepts of self, world, and motivation.* In order to elicit the child's view of himself and his cosmology and understand his motivational styles, the following may be probed:

  a. self-concept descriptions, self-demands,

  b. expectations of future events and role in effecting change,

  c. daydreams, and

  d. fantasy material and special fairy tales.

6. *Mood and affective expression.* It goes without saying that any comprehensive assessment battery should include a rating of pervasive mood and its predominant mode of expression. This may present a problem, especially in the case of "younger" children who might not be able to self-report or who may label their affective states inaccurately.

7. *Biochemical and biophysiological variables.* The presently existing methodologies employed in the study of biochemical and other physiological aspects of adult depressive illnesses may also be used with youngsters where indicated.

The committee felt that the scales must also take into account a time dimension. It was recommended that assessments be made for current status in conjunction with obtaining a developmental psychiatric history.

In many cases the content of the measurement instruments is inextricably tied to the manner in which the data are gathered. This is especially true with younger children, in whom observational methods go hand in hand with objectively ratable overt behavior. Keeping in mind that the appropriateness of some of the following is determined by the child's age, the committee discussed these data-gathering approaches:

1. *Observational methods.* The development of rating scales to facilitate the systematic assessment of overt, observable behavior

should be a priority. The measurement of depression among younger children is likely to rely heavily on such observational methods.

2. *Self-rating/self-description.* This type of assessment may be implemented in at least two ways. One avenue involves the development of novel self-rating scales, based, for example, on data gathered by the methods outlined in strategies A through D. Another avenue is to start with currently existing self-rating scales for adult depression. Such scales may be modified with respect to reading grade level and age-appropriate content areas.

3. *Ratings/descriptions of the subject by others.* It is recommended that rating scales be geared toward adults whose roles *vis-à-vis* the child assure different perspectives. In addition to clinicians' rating scales, scales should be used with parents as well as teachers (when appropriate). As in the case of self-ratings, the scales may be adaptations of currently existing scales used with depressed adults. Such scales may then, in turn, be modified in terms of language, content, and specificity for use with parents and teachers. The data-gathering procedures outlined in strategies A through D may also yield relevant information as to content areas and behaviors that such scales should cover.

Raters

Traditionally, clinical syndromes have been assessed through self-ratings/self-descriptions and through descriptions and assessment by clinicians. The committee recommended that the utility of nonclinically trained professional as well as "lay" raters be explored. Thus, a multifaceted assessment approach should make provisions for ratings by parents, teachers, and pediatricians.

Sampling Problems

The committee felt that sampling problems vary according to how the index cases are defined and the particular research questions asked. If the youngsters themselves are the index cases, they may be initially defined in terms of absence or assumed presence of depressive pathology. Another strategy might involve defining parents as index cases either in terms of overt depressive symptomatology or in terms of the assumed potential of their status for engendering depression in their children (e.g., terminal illness).

The committee felt that in younger children, sampling problems are accentuated by the general inaccessibility of the age group as research subjects. It was felt that in addition to the clearly accessible in- or outpatient populations of child guidance centers, collaborative arrangements with pediatricians would greatly enhance the likelihood of locating children with some form of psychological difficulties. Thus, depending on the design employed to study childhood depression the samples may be: (1) standard pediatric/school subjects, (2) pediatric/school subjects selected for some symptomatology, (3) psychiatric in- or outpatient subjects selected or unselected for depressive symptomatology, and (4) children of adult index cases.

Study Designs

The committee recognized that the description and assessment of childhood depression may be approached through a number of different routes.

To be precise, these approaches would qualify only as "pre-experimental" or at best "quasi-experimental" designs. The committee felt that among other possible avenues, the following represent feasible and potentially fruitful approaches:

1. *One-shot case comparison studies* (e.g., contrasting psychiatric and normal subjects or various groups of psychiatric subjects; prevalence studies).

2. *Cross-sectional developmental studies* (e.g., comparing, at any one point in time, prevalence and characteristics of the syndrome among different age groups of normal and psychiatric subjects).

3. *Longitudinal follow-up or comparison studies* (e.g., follow-up of children of adult index cases, comparison of pediatric "problem" and normal cases over time, follow-up of various child psychiatric samples).

RECOMMENDED RESEARCH QUESTIONS

As a possible direction for future research, the committee formulated a number of potentially viable research questions in the context of which the description and assessment of childhood depression may be pursued. These questions are phrased in general ways and are intended as potential guidelines.

1. Question: What are the symptom characteristics and duration of normally occurring adjustment reactions in response to major life events among children of different age groups?

Method: Define "adjustment event" *a priori* as an event with a high likelihood to require an adjustment with possible depressive elements (for example, impending death of a terminally ill parent or postpartum psychosis of the mother). Study these children with respect to multiplicity and duration of symptoms.

2. Question: Are somatic problems in childhood indicative of subsequent depressions?

Method: Select very young pediatric samples with some target

symptoms such as excessive weepiness, "colicyness," or feeding disturbances, and a sample of nonproblem pediatric controls. Follow these groups to assess their psychiatric status at
ages 8 or 12.

3. Question: What is the prevalence of depressive symptoms in
"normal" and "psychiatric" child populations?

Method: Apply the depression assessment battery to selected
groups of "psychiatric" and "nonpsychiatric" populations to
ascertain differential base rates of occurrence of depressive
symptoms.

4. Question: Do the results of a depression assessment battery
enhance differential diagnosis among a group of child psychiatric
cases?

Method: Systematically evaluate large groups of child psychiatric in- and outpatients irrespective of presenting problem or
reason for hospitalization. Ascertain if the assessment data
discriminate among various groups especially with respect to
presenting problem.

5. Question: Does the presence of a clinically depressed parent
engender depression in a child?

Method: Evaluate children of clinically depressed mothers and
compare them to children of equivalent nondepressed psychiatric controls.

6. Question: Do "high-risk" children manifest early signs of
depressive illness?

Method: In "genetically biased" populations such as the children of manic-depressive parents, assess their behavior compared to that of control children (controlling for the effects of
parental hospitalizations, if any).

7. Question: Do youngsters diagnosed by the extensive assessment battery as depressed show differential responses to antidepressant, antianxiety, or placebo medication?

Method: Randomly assign to the three treatment modalities a
large sample of children unequivocally diagnosed as depressed
by the assessment battery. Assess their responses to medication. (Note: although antidepressants are apparently extensively
used in youngsters, their efficacy in the treatment of clear-cut
childhood depressions has not been unequivocally
demonstrated.)

8. Question: What is the relationship between major familial life
events and children's behavioral responses?

Method: Ascertain whether differing major familial life events,
such as divorce, death of a parent, or birth of a sibling, serve as
precipitating factors for depressive versus other responses.

SUMMARY AND OVERALL RECOMMENDATIONS

The general sentiment of the committee was that childhood depressive disorders are "real" clinical phenomena and that rigorous clinical and empirical investigations of this area are needed.

It was also felt that clinically oriented investigations of normal development are essential. Such investigations can provide normative data against which the assumed validity of psychological symptoms and syndromes can be assessed.

Clinical description and psychometric assessment of childhood depressions was seen as a first step in bringing order to this diffuse area. Subsequent to the development of a good assessment battery that can discriminate depressed from nondepressed children, a look at clustering of symptoms and subclassification would be worthwhile. Further analysis based on classifying children with respect to precipitating events may also be fruitful.

Epidemiological studies may be used to test the validity of any criterion purported to define depression. For example, if an epidemiological study of normal youngsters discloses a very high prevalence of the symptoms under consideration, a redefinition on the original criteria might well be indicated.

Finally, the committee felt that a thorough assessment and understanding of clinical phenomenology is needed if efforts at subclassification or effective treatment modalities are to be worthwhile. It was strongly recommended that research be carried out on cases over an extended period of time, and that normal developmental variations be distinguished from clinical depression. Last but not least, there was a strong sentiment that, at this point, assessment and research into childhood depressions are most likely to benefit from an emphasis on actual rather than inferred behaviors.

Depression in Childhood: Diagnosis, Treatment, and Conceptual Models, edited by J. G. Schulterbrandt and A. Raskin. Raven Press, New York, 1977.

Report of Subcommittee on the Treatment of Depression in Children

Judith L. Rapoport, Chairperson

The Committee on Treatment was faced with a dilemma about what we were supposed to treat. We spent some time discussing the prematurity of treatment without syndrome identification, even if used as a means of identifying subgroups of depressed children.

Our clearest recommendation for the preadolescent age group is that we are rather specifically not recommending that the NIMH fund any large treatment program at the moment because that would be premature. This does not mean that some small pilot studies might not be undertaken. For example, an investigator might select a group of children with headaches or learning problems thought to be secondary to depression and treat them with an antidepressant drug. Such a study could be funded by the NIMH, but certainly this is not the time to make the treatment of depression in children a major priority.

Dr. Anthony presented some data from two groups of children, ages 9 to 11 and 12 to 14, from a general child psychiatric clinic. All of the children had school failure, but he felt that only a small percentage of these groups would have fulfilled the criteria for depression he outlined, which included dysphoric mood, low self-esteem, and drastic mood change.

When Dr. Anthony and others on the committee considered populations of children with known organic brain damage, it was felt that there was a much higher incidence, perhaps 20 or 30%, of such clinic populations showing signs of "depression."

One issue we couldn't dodge was that drug treatment of children was a fact of life—particularly among pediatricians. Hence, one positive recommendation was that a survey be implemented to determine what therapies pediatricians and child psychiatrists are currently using. Emphasis in such a survey might be placed on what drug therapies are being used for children with psychological and psychiatric problems other than hyperactivity or psychosis.

It was also our pooled impression that there is currently a wide use of drug treatment for anxiety and psychosomatic symptoms of childhood. If this widespread use were documented, it might be advisable to have some rigorously controlled drug efficacy studies either to correct or to confirm current practices. For example, there is a good deal of use by pediatricians of minor tranquilizers for children with anxiety symptoms.

The final recommendation we discussed was the possibility of some small pilot studies of masked depression that might examine therapy in relation to genetic background or biochemical measures.

Subject Index

Abdominal pain
  as characteristic in depressive phobic
    anxiety state, 6
  as depressive symptom, 5, 50
  as masked depressive symptom, 9, 52
Abnormal behavior in primates, rehabilita-
    tion of, 119–120
Abraham study (1968), on theoretical child-
    hood depression, 17
Accident proneness, as masked depressive
    symptom, 8
Acting-out
  by depressive children, 54–56
  as object-loss anxiety/despair, 54
  psychodynamic and social meanings of,
    55
  as sign of depression, 51
Adolescence
  absence of depression before, 137–138
  hyperactivity symptoms in, 92
Adolescents, special problems and treat-
    ment for, 27–31
Adrenal catecholamine-synthesizing
    enzymes, mother-infant separation
    reaction as inducing, 118
Adrenal tyrosine hydrolase, level-elevations
    in, as induced by mother-infant separa-
    tion reaction, 119
Affect reversals, as sign of depression, 51
Affectional systems in rhesus monkey, 112–
    113
Affectual depression, incidence common in
    6- to 8-year-olds, 3
African parrot, separation studies on, 108
Age
  affectual depression common in 6- to 8-
    year-olds, 3
  in assessment approaches, 155
  in depressive proneness, 36
  in deviant behavior, 141, 145
  guilt depression frequent after year 11, 3
  and language as communicator after
    seventh year, 2
  in mood variability, 144
  in mother-infant separation reactions,
    115, 116
  negative self-esteem depression in 8- to
    11-year-olds, 3
Aggression
  to avoid depressed feelings, 55
  as depressive symptom, 4–5, 71
  difficulties in handling, as reason for
    referral, 51
  and headache, as depressive symptom, 94
  and hyperactivity, stimulant effects on,
    88–89
  internalized, in latency-age depression, 49
  among males, higher incidence of, 96
  as masked depressive symptom, 8–10

repressed, as leading to depression, 39
  against self, as masochistic phenomena,
    49
Agitated behavior, as depressive symptom,
    3
Alexander, Franz, on neurotic-character
    model, 54
Aloneness, as factor in mother-infant
    separation response, 116
Alpha-methyl-paratyrosine (AMPT)
  and depletion of brain amines, 118
  dosages that affect behavioral changes,
    118
  and placebo effects on peer-separation
    reaction, 117
Altruism, related to masochism and self-
    pity, 52
Ambivalence
  toward love object, as depressive
    symptom, 70
  toward maternal-role bearer, in de-
    pression, 40
Amitriptyline, see also Antidepressant
    treatment; Tricyclics
  early-morning waking as indication for,
    102
  efficacy of, in Lucas study, 96
Amphetamines, see also Stimulants
  and increased cortical inhibition, 101
  side effects of, 101–102, 104, 148
  as stimulants, effects on children vs.
    adults, 88–89
Anger
  necessity of, 45
  outbursts of, as masked depressive
    symptom, 9
  relationship to guilt, 46
  role of, in depressive response, 41
Anhedonia
  as depressive symptom, 73, 79, 141
  as diagnostic criteria, 141, 153
Animal behavioral/biological models
  abnormal behavior in, rehabilitation of,
    119–120
  advantages of, 109–110, 120
  of depressive/affective disorders, 107–120
  development of, four major areas in, 109
  induction techniques in, 109
  nonacceptance of, grounds for, 107
  potential uses for, 116
  rationale for using, 108
  study of underlying neurobiological
    mechanisms in, 110
Annell studies (1969, 1972)
  on lithium use in children/adolescents,
    96–97
  on lithium treatment with mixed diag-
    nostic categories, 102–103
Anorexia